NURSING AND THE CHILDBEARING FAMILY: A Guide for Study

DEBRA P. HYMOVICH, R.N., B.S., M.A.

Associate Professor, University of Texas
Clinical Nursing School at San Antonio

SUELLEN B. REED, R.N., B.S.N., M.S.N.

Assistant Professor, The University of Texas
Clinical Nursing School at San Antonio

1971

W. B. SAUNDERS COMPANY • PHILADELPHIA • LONDON • TORONTO

W. B. Saunders Company: West Washington Square
Philadelphia, Pa. 19105

12 Dyott Street
London, WC1A 1DB

1835 Yonge Street
Toronto 7, Ontario

Nursing and the Childbearing Family: A Guide for Study SBN 0-7216-4956-4

 Made in the United States of America. Press of W. B. Saunders Company. Library of Congress catalog card number 76-151679.

Print No: 9 8 7 6 5 4 3 2 1

This book is dedicated
by
Debra P. Hymovich
TO HER MOTHER, LILLIAN HYMOVICH,
and by
Suellen B. Reed
TO HER PARENTS, JOHN W. AND MARY E. BRENNER

PREFACE

These study guides have been written to provide a framework within which students can begin to discover areas in which nursing can assist families during childbearing and the beginning phases of childrearing. The guides are designed to involve the nursing student in her own learning by having her select information needed to propose solutions to nursing problems. Emphasis is placed on the anticipatory guidance role of the nurse in promoting a high level of wellness for all members of the family. The student is guided in understanding herself, in determining knowledge needed for her nursing role, and in becoming aware of current social issues related to the childbearing family.

The study guides are designed to:

1. Stimulate the student by encouraging personal discovery;
2. Involve the student in her own learning by proposing solutions to nursing problems involving childbearing families;
3. Guide the student in acquiring knowledge applicable to nursing from a variety of disciplines;
4. Guide the student in using the nursing process of assessment, planning, implementation and evaluation of care in a variety of situations related to childbearing;
5. Encourage creative problem solving based on scientific knowledge;
6. Encourage critical thinking.

Each guide is designed to stand alone, or parts of several guides may be selected to be used concurrently in providing a different emphasis for study. The guides may be used in preparation for or to augment classes and/or the clinical practicum.

The two assessment guides can be used by students when caring for members of childbearing families in a variety of settings.

Nurses in hospital settings have limited contact with families during their childbearing experiences. It is the nurse in the community who can influence primary prevention of untoward experiences among these families. Therefore, these guides are relevant to nursing students in the community aspects of their professional programs.

Many of these study guides show the progression of the Wonder family through an essentially normal childbearing experience. This family can be used as a thread of continuity throughout a given course even though all students are not having the same clinical practicum. Other study guides include selected aspects of the course of pregnancy, labor, delivery and postpartal care of high risk women, their infants and their families.

Material for consideration is presented at the point in time, in so far as possible, at which it has the most significance for nursing and/or medical care. For example, pelvic measurements are generally obtained early in pregnancy, but the implications are related to the labor and delivery process. Thus, pelvimetry is included in the guide related to Amy Wonder's labor and delivery.

The references at the end of each study guide have been selected because of their relevance to the questions in the guide and for the bibliographies which they provide for the student or instructor who would like to refer to the original sources or pursue a topic in more depth. The references have been selected from a variety of sources and there may be several references to one topic so as to serve the needs of the student who has access to a limited library.

The annotations following some of the references serve to clarify the content of those articles whose titles are not self-explanatory.

The student is encouraged to seek knowledge from a variety of sources and to critically evaluate all she sees, hears and reads. With an understanding of the knowledge, research and trends in nursing and related fields, nurses can contribute a high quality of professional nursing care to childbearing families.

DEBRA P. HYMOVICH
SUELLEN B. REED

ACKNOWLEDGMENTS

We wish to acknowledge the assistance of the following people in the preparation of this study guide:

- Sandra King, Assistant Professor, University of Texas Clinical Nursing School, San Antonio, Texas
- Linda Lambert, Assistant Professor, University of Arkansas School of Nursing, Little Rock, Arkansas
- Nancy Maebius, Instructor, University of Texas Clinical Nursing School, San Antonio, Texas
- Susan McCabe, Instructor, University of Florida College of Nursing, Gainesville, Florida
- The nursing students who have used and tested these guides
- Judy Davis for her typing of this manuscript

D.P.H.
S.B.R.

CONTENTS

Guide 1

INTRODUCTION TO NURSING OF CHILDBEARING FAMILIES

PART I. THE FAMILY

Nursing care of a woman during her childbearing years must include care of her entire family if it is to be comprehensive and is to promote a high level of wellness. This study guide will introduce you to concepts which should be applied in the family situation study guides which follow.

1. State the meaning of the following terms used in reference to providing nursing health services to childbearing families.

   a. Maternity nursing

   b. Obstetrical nursing

   c. Maternal and infant nursing

d. Maternal and child nursing

e. Family nursing

f. Nurse midwifery

2. State the meaning of the following terms used to describe a family constellation.

   a. Nuclear family

   b. Extended family

   c. Communal family

3. The family is referred to as a social system. What components of a social system have application to the family unit?

4. How can knowledge of the family constellation be used by the nurse in providing care for a childbearing family?

5. Developmental tasks have been identified for the family as well as for the various stages of growth and development from infancy through adulthood.

   a. What is a developmental task?

   b. How can the nurse use knowledge of developmental tasks in providing care to childbearing families?

6. On the chart below:

   a. State one developmental task for each of the following families:

      1) Beginning family (establishment phase)

      2) Expectant family

      3) The childbearing family (with infant or toddler)

      4) Family with preschool children

5) Family with school children

6) Family with teenagers

b. For each task, state:

1) At least two occurrences or situations which would promote attainment of the task and a cohesive family unit

2) Two occurrences which would inhibit attainment of the task

FAMILY	*TASK*	*PROMOTE ATTAINMENT*	*INHIBIT ATTAINMENT*

7. Knowledge of family socioeconomic class is basic to effectively providing for the delivery of nursing health services to the childbearing family.

   a. State some of your beliefs about the characteristics of members of the following:

      1) Lower social class

      2) Middle social class

      3) Upper social class

   b. The chart below lists come of the areas which need to be considered by nurses in relation to family social class. State the information needed to complete this chart for the lower, middle and upper social classes in relation to the areas listed in the first column.

AREAS OF CONSIDERATION	*LOWER SOCIAL CLASS*	*MIDDLE SOCIAL CLASS*	*UPPER SOCIAL CLASS*
Income range			
Average family size			

AREAS OF CONSIDERATION	*LOWER SOCIAL CLASS*	*MIDDLE SOCIAL CLASS*	*UPPER SOCIAL CLASS*
Usual educational level			
Nutritional status			
Significance of the family			
Self image			
Family planning			
Plans for future			
Beliefs about health and health care			
Type of health care facilities used			

8. Select from the previous chart at least four of the areas to be considered by nurses in relation to family social class. For each of the areas you have selected, state at least two nursing implications which are relevant to the childbearing family in each social class (lower, middle, and upper).

	NURSING IMPLICATIONS		
AREA	*LOWER CLASS*	*MIDDLE CLASS*	*UPPER CLASS*

9. How do you think your beliefs and your social class background will influence your nursing care of childbearing families?

10. An understanding of cultural differences is basic to providing individualized nursing services for childbearing families. Select one culture other than your own and state:

    a. Three characteristics or beliefs of the culture which are related to childbearing

b. The nursing implications of each of these characteristics or beliefs

11. The nurse must be aware of the influence of religion on the beliefs and practices of the childbearing family. Compare two different religions by stating specific examples of how the religious beliefs and practices might influence the childbearing family.

12. How do you think your religious background may influence your nursing care of childbearing families?

13. Anticipatory guidance is a necessary component of the nursing services needed by childbearing families.

a. What is anticipatory guidance?

b. Suggest three areas in which anticipatory guidance would be useful to:

1) Teenagers prior to marriage

2) Beginning families (from marriage until pregnancy)

3) Expectant families

14. Explain how your attitudes and feelings may influence the care you give families during their childbearing experiences.

15. The nurse needs to assess the childbearing family with whom she is working in order to make realistic and individualized nursing care plans with the family.

    a. What is a nursing assessment?

    b. State the skills you need in order to perform a nursing assessment.

16. For each of the four areas listed below, state:

    a. The information which would be useful to nurses working with childbearing families

    b. How this information might be used in planning and providing nursing care

        1) Health status of family members

        2) Previous health care

3) Family's expectations regarding health and health care

4) Home environment

5) Educational background

6) Family constellation

PART II. ASSESSMENT GUIDE: RESPONSE TO CHILDBEARING

This may be used as a guide when you are assessing members of childbearing families in order to plan nursing intervention.

A. Significant data related to person's health:

1. Previous health care (for what, where, when, reaction to it)

2. Woman's and family's expectations regarding health and health care:

   (a) Present

   (b) Future

B. Significant data related to childbearing:

1. Woman's and family's understanding of conception, pregnancy, labor and delivery and child care

2. Physiological alterations of childbearing (antepartal or postpartal periods) and management of alterations:

   Changes in body and body function including:

   Configuration

   Skin

   Weight

   Breasts

   Rest and sleep

   Posture

   Mobility

   Breathing

Eating

Elimination

Senses

Vagina and uterus

Vascular system

3. Psychosocial changes of childbearing (antepartal and postpartal periods), and management of changes:

Changes in psychosocial activities including:

Mood

Temperament

Feelings toward pregnancy and baby

Dependence and independence

Relationships with others

Recreation

Employment

C. Significant data related to family living:

1. Plans for home care of:

(a) Mother

(b) Infant

(c) Other family members

2. Family preparation for new member

3. Other (such as health or environmental consideration)

REFERENCES

BOOKS

Anthony, E. J., and Benedek, T. (Eds.): *Parenthood; its Psychology and Psychopathology.* Boston, Little Brown and Company, 1970.

Barnes, A. C.: "Prevention of Congenital Anomalies from the Point of View of the Obstetrician." *Congenital Malformations.* International Medical Congress, Ltd., 1964. (Genetic counseling; prenatal care; maternal disease; pregnancy-related diseases; labor and delivery.)

Barron, M. L. (Ed.): *Minorities in a Changing World.* New York, Alfred A. Knopf, 1967.

Benson, L.: *Fatherhood – A Sociological Perspective.* New York, Random House, 1968.

Brown, M. I.: "Implications of Cultural Change for Maternal and Child Health Nursing." *Culture, Atmosphere and Social Organization: Effects on Nursing Care of the Patient,* pp. 18-33. ANA Clinical Sessions, 10 Columbus Circle, New York, 1962. (Maternal and child health practices of Puerto Rican-born women in New York City; implications of nursing.)

Cavan, R. S.: *The American Family.* 4th Ed., pp. 1-20, 71-84. New York, Thomas Y. Crowell Company, 1969. (Characteristics of the American Family; social class, ethnic groups.)

Clausen, J. A.: "Family Structure, Socialization and Personality." In Hoffman, L. W., and Hoffman, M. L.: *Review of Child Development Research.* Vol. 2. New York, Russell Sage Foundation, 1966.

Duvall, E. M.: *Family Development.* 3rd Ed. Philadelphia, J. B. Lippincott Company, 1971.

Feldman, F. L., and Scherz, F. H.: *Family Social Welfare,* pp. 63-72. New York, Atherton Press, 1967. (Definitions of family; nuclear and extended families; roles of family members; family tasks, cycle of family life.)

Hess, R. D.: "Social Class and Ethnic Influences Upon Socialization." In Mussen, P. H.: *Carmichael's Manual of Child Psychology.* New York, John Wiley and Sons, Inc., 1970.

Hurlock, E. B.: *Developmental Psychology.* 3rd Ed. New York, McGraw-Hill Book Company, 1968.

Nordmark, M. T., and Rohweder, A. W.: *Scientific Foundations of Nursing.* 2nd Ed., pp. 323-329. Philadelphia, J. B. Lippincott Company, 1967.

Pohlman, E., and Pohlman, J. M.: *The Psychology of Birth Planning.* Cambridge, Massachusetts, Schenkman Publishing Company, Inc., 1969. (The desire for children; costs of conception; husband-wife relationships; parental roles; unwanted conceptions and parents' feelings; methods of birth planning; psychological aspects of overpopulation.)

Wray, J. D.: *The Population Explosion and the Family.* Chapel Hill, North Carolina, University of North Carolina Press, 1968.

JOURNAL ARTICLES

Baca, J. E.: "Some Health Beliefs of the Spanish Speaking." *American Journal of Nursing,* 69:2172, October 1969. (Beliefs and practices of Spanish-Americans regarding health and illness.)

Berkowitz, P., and Berkowitz, N. S.: "The Jewish Patient in the Hospital." *American Journal of Nursing,* 67:2335, November 1967. (Basic beliefs of Judaism.)

Collins, R. D.: "Problem Solving – a Tool for Patients, Too." *American Journal of Nursing,* 68:1483, July 1968. (Process of problem solving; helping patients with process.)

Costello, D. E.: "Communication Patterns in Family Systems." *Nursing Clinics of North America,* 4:721, December 1969.

Drapela, V. J.: "Personality Adjustment and Religious Growth." *Religion and Health,* 8:87, January 1969.

Elder, G. H., Jr., and Bowerman, C. E.: "Family Structure and Childrearing Patterns: The Effect of Family Size and Sex Composition." *American Sociological Review,* 28:891, 1963.

Francis, G. M.: "How Do I Feel about Myself?" *American Journal of Nursing,* 67:1244, June 1967.

Goldstein, J.: "Exploring Attitudes that Affect Nursing Care." *Nursing Outlook,* 16:50, June 1968. (Attitudes of practical nursing students toward death and birth.)

Haggerty, R. J.: "Family Diagnosis: Research Methods and Their Reliability for Studies of the Medical-Social Unit, the Family." *American Journal of Public Health,* 55:1521, October 1965.

Herzog, E., and Lewis, H.: "Children in Poor Families: Myths and Realities." *American Journal of Orthopsychiatry,* 40:375, April 1970.

Kearns, B. J. R.: "Childrearing Practices among Selected Culturally Deprived Minorities." *The Journal of Genetic Psychology,* 116:149, June 1970.

Leininger, M. M.: "Nursing Care of a Patient from Another Culture." *Nursing Clinics of North America,* 2:747, December 1967. (Significance of culture and human behavior to nursing; the Japanese-American patient.)

Loughlin, B. W.: "Pregnancy in the Navajo Culture." *Nursing Outlook,* 13:55, March 1965.

McCain, F. R.: "Nursing by Assessment – Not Intuition,"*American Journal of Nursing,* 65:82, April 1965.

Mead, M.: "The Changing American Family." *Children,* 10:173, September-October 1963.

Muecke, M. A.: "Overcoming the Language Barrier." *Nursing Outlook,* 18:53, April 1970. (Ways of communicating with people who cannot or do not speak your language.)

Murray, J. B.: "Self-Knowledge and the Nursing Interview." *Nursing Forum,* 11:1:69, 1963. (Nurses' self-understanding and acceptance as basic to any interaction with patients.)

Porter, E. R.: "From Mountain Folk to City Dwellers." *Nursing Outlook,* 11:514, July 1963. (Some characteristics of Southern Appalachian migrants and suggestions for working with them.)

Richie, J.: "Using an Interpreter Effectively." *Nursing Outlook,* 12:27, December 1964. (A guide to avoiding mishaps and misunderstandings.)

Robischon, P., and Scott, D.: "Role Theory and its Application in Family Nursing." *Nursing Outlook,* 17:52, July 1969.

Sussman, M. B., and Burchinal, L. G.: "Parental Aid to Married Children: Implications for Family Functioning." *Marriage and Family Living,* 24:320, 1962.

Tallman, I.: "The Family as a Small Problem Solving Group." *Journal of Marriage and the Family,* 32:94, February 1970.

Vander Zanden, J. W.: "The Minority Group Patient." *Nursing Outlook,* 12:57, February 1964. (Reactions of minority group members include accommodation, avoidance, aggression, hypersensitivity, ego-enhancement and self-hatred.)

Vander Zanden, J. W., and Vander Zanden, M. V.: "The Interview." *Nursing Outlook,* 11:743, October 1963. (What questions to ask and how.)

Watts, W.: "Social Class, Ethnic Background and Patient Care." *Nursing Forum,* 6:2:155, 1967. (Beliefs of lower and middle socioeconomic classes, whites and nonwhites.)

Yeaworth, R. C.: "Students' Attitudes Toward Maternal Role." *Nursing Outlook,* 15:37, July 1967. (Influence of preconceived ideas on students' relationships with maternity patients.)

Zimmerman, D. S. and Gohrke, C.: "The Goal-Directed Nursing Approach." *American Journal of Nursing,* 70:306, February 1970.

OTHER PUBLICATIONS

Cahill, I. D.: "The Mother from the Slum Neighborhood." *(Conference on Maternal and Child Nursing: Current Concepts in Nursing Care.)* Columbus, Ohio, Ross Laboratories, 1964.

Irelan, L. M. (Ed.): *Low-Income Life Styles.* Washington, D.C., U.S. Department of Health, Education, and Welfare, 1967. (Goals and values; life themes; family patterns; education; health practices.)

NOTES

Guide 2

HEALTH AND THE CHILDBEARING FAMILY

1. Why is it important for nurses to be aware of the trends in morbidity and mortality related to the childbearing family?

2. The following terms are used in presenting vital statistics related to childbearing families. For each of the terms listed on the chart below, state:

   a. Its meaning

   b. The current rate

   c. The trend in the United States

   d. Factors influencing this trend

TERMS	*MEANING*	*RATE*	*TREND*	*FACTORS INFLUENCING TREND*
Live birth rate				
Fetal mortality rate				
Neonatal mortality rate				
Infant mortality rate				
Perinatal mortality rate				
Maternal mortality rate				

3. State the leading causes in the United States of the following:

   a. Infant deaths

b. Premature infant deaths

c. Maternal deaths

4. a. State how the United States compares with other countries in terms of:

   1) Neonatal mortality

   2) Maternal mortality

   b. What significance does this have for the health professions?

5. Many women in the United States do not receive adequate prenatal care.

   a. State the reasons why many women do not receive adequate prenatal care.

b. State the implications this has for nursing. Be specific.

6. State the contributions of the following types of nurses to the delivery of health services to childbearing families.

a. Nurses in labor, delivery and postpartal units of the hospital

b. Nurses in a maternity clinic or physician's office

c. Nurses in a community (public health) setting

d. Inactive nurses at home raising a family

7. Genetic counseling is becoming an important aspect of preconceptional care.

   a. What is genetic counseling?

   b. Why is genetic counseling necessary?

   c. What is the physician's role in genetic counseling?

   d. What is the nurse's role in genetic counseling?

8. a. What percentage of childbearing women and their infants are considered high risk?

   b. What is meant by high risk?

c. What factors contribute to a pregnancy's becoming high risk?

d. What factors contribute to an infant's being classified as high risk?

9. Many agencies play a role in fostering good maternity and infant care. Why is it important for nurses to be familiar with the resources these agencies have to offer?

10. Briefly state the contribution each of the following resources makes toward maternal and infant care.

    a. Maternity Center Association

b. Office of Child Development (Children's Bureau)

c. Maternal and Infant Care Programs

d. La Leche League

e. American Academy of Obstetrics and Gynecology

f. American Nurses' Association

g. National League for Nursing

h. Academy of Pediatrics

i. National Institutes of Neurological Diseases and Blindness

j. National Red Cross

k. White House Conferences for Children and Youth

11. Delivery of health care services to childbearing families is inadequate at the present time.

    a. Identify several of the current problems related to the provision of health services to childbearing families.

    b. Suggest at least one solution for each problem you have identified.

12. What implications do these current problems and possible solutions in the delivery of health services to childbearing families have for the expanded role of the family nurse?

REFERENCES

BOOKS

American Academy of Pediatrics: *Standards and Recommendations for Hospital Care of Newborn Infants.* Evanston, Illinois, The American Academy of Pediatrics, 1964.

American Public Health Association: *Infant, Perinatal, Maternal, and Childhood Mortality in the United States.* Cambridge, Massachusetts, Harvard University Press, 1968. (Trends and recent status; factors influencing infant and perinatal trends; international comparisons; health services and resources.)

Barnes, A. C.: "Prevention of Congenital Anomalies from the Point of View of the Obstetrician." *Congenital Malformations.* International Medical Congress, Limited, 1964. (Genetic counseling; prenatal care; maternal disease; pregnancy-related diseases; labor and delivery.)

Bryant, R. D., and Overland, A. E.: *Obstetric Management and Nursing.* 7th Ed. Philadelphia, F. A. Davis Company, 1964. (Baptism.)

Fishbein, M. (Ed.): *Birth Defects.* Philadelphia, J. B. Lippincott Company, 1963. (Genetic counseling.)

Haselkorn, F. (Ed.): *Mothers-at-Risk.* New York, Adelphi University School of Social Work, 1966. (Problems; characteristics; policies; services for high risk mothers.)

Kenneth, H. Y.: "Community Nursing Service to the 'Well Family'." In *ANA Clinical Sessions,* pp. 72-79. New York, Appleton-Century-Crofts, 1968. (Role developed by one nurse as she worked with one family.)

Lerch, C.: *Maternity Nursing.* St. Louis, The C. V. Mosby Company, 1970.

Lidz, T.: *The Person; His Development Throughout the Life Cycle.* pp. 45-69. New York, Basic Books, Inc., 1968. (The family.)

Manual of Standards in Obstetric-Gynecologic Practice. 2nd Ed. Chicago, The American College of Obstetricians and Gynecologists, 1965. (p. 25, lay education; pp. 104-108, definitions.)

The Midwife in the United States. New York, Josiah Macy, Jr. Foundation, 1968. (Includes personnel needs in maternity care; training and role of midwives in U.S.; midwives in other countries; development of new patterns of care and new types of personnel for maternal and child health.)

O'Connell, E.: "Hospital Maternity Nursing – Then and Now." In Bergersen, B. S., at al. (Eds.): *Current Concepts in Clinical Nursing.* Vol. 2, Chapter 30. St. Louis, The C. V. Mosby Company, 1969. (Compares maternity nursing care of the 1930's and 1940's with that of the late 1960's by using patient care situations.)

Stevenson, A. C.: *Genetic Counseling.* Philadelphia, J. B. Lippincott Company, 1970. (Introduction.)

Vital Statistics of the United States. Washington, D.C., U.S. Department of Health, Education and Welfare. (Current volumes.)

Whipple, D. V.: *Dynamics of Human Development.* Euthenic Pediatrics, pp. 18-29. New York, McGraw-Hill Book Company, 1966. (Mortality rates, causes.)

JOURNAL ARTICLES

Anderson, E. H., and Lesser, A. J.: "Maternity Care in the United States, Gains and Gaps." *American Journal of Nursing,* 66:1539, July 1966. (Statistical data, legislation – overview from 1915 to 1966.)

Apgar, V., and Stickle, G.: "Birth Defects." *Journal of the American Medical Association,* 204:371, April 29, 1968. (Definition and taxonomy; fetal loss; prevalence.)

Apone, J.: "Children of Society's Ills." *American Journal of Nursing,* 66:1750, August 1966. (Conditions of minority group patients in the United States.)

Bartsch, V.: "Standardization of Terminology, Reporting of Live Births, Fetal Deaths." *Hospital Topics,* 46:97, February 1968. (Birth certificate; fetal death certificate.)

Bartuska, D. G.: "Genetic Counseling." *Clinical Obstetrics and Gynecology,* 9:699, September 1966.

Berman, J.: "Some Things Learned." *American Journal of Public Health and the Nation's Health,* 59:930, June 1969. (Maternal child health and public health; an overview in prevention.)

Buchsbaum, H. J.: "Accidental Injury Complicating Pregnancy." *American Journal of Obstetrics and Gynecology,* 102:752, November 1, 1968.

Chase, H. C.: "Perinatal and Infant Mortality in the United States and Six West European Countries." *American Journal of Public Health,* 57:1735, October 1967. (Comparative study 1950 to 1964; trends; causes of death; possible future trends.)

Downs, F. S.: "Maternal Stress in Primigravidas as a Factor in the Production of Neonatal Pathology." *Nursing Science,* 2:348, October 1964. (Reviews causes of perinatal morbidity and mortality; report of research to investigate relationship between maternal stress and neonatal pathology.)

Drage, J. S., et al.: "The Apgar Score as an Index of Neonatal Mortality." *Obstetrics and Gynecology,* 24:222, August 1964.

Edwards, J.: "Needed: Patient-Oriented Nursing in the Maternity Unit." *Hospital Topics,* 48:83, March 1970. (Emphasizes and explains "maternal nursing.")

Falkner, F.: "Infant Mortality, an Urgent National Problem." *Children,* 17:83, May-June 1970. (Mortality rates in U.S.; priorities for improvement.)

Forbes, N. P.: "The Nurse and Genetic Counseling." *Nursing Clinics of North America,* 1:679, December 1966. (Chromosomal and genetic errors; genetic clinic services; nurse's role.)

Gold, E. M.: "Identification of the High Risk Fetus." *Clinical Obstetrics and Gynecology,* 11:1069, December 1968. (Assessment of infant mortality and morbidity; criteria for identifying high risk pregnancy and high risk infant; application of criteria.)

Gold, E. M., and Stone, M. L.: "Total Maternal and Infant Care: A Realistic Appraisal." *American Journal of Public Health,* 58:1219, July 1968. (Care including home visits, prenatal, postpartal and infant care, patient education, nutrition services.)

Gray, J. W.: "Liaison Nurses Bridge the Care Gap." *Nursing Outlook,* 15:28, May 1967. (Nurses act as liaison for high risk maternity patients between clinic, hospital, and community.)

Hennel, M.: "Family-Centered Maternity Nursing in Practice." *Nursing Clinics of North America,* 3:289, June 1968. (Stresses maternity care as including high school students; pre-Cana conferences, clinics, hospital and home; includes aspects of teaching that include fathers.)

Hilliard, M. E.: "The Evaluation of a Maternity Nurse." *Nursing Forum,* IV:2:6, 1965. (Changes in maternity nursing; considerations for the future.)

Hilliard, M. E.: "New Horizons in Maternity Nursing." *Nursing Outlook,* 15:33, July 1967. (Description of what happens to a woman during antepartal, intrapartal and postpartal periods; implications for role of nurse.)

Hilmar, N.: "Standards and Criteria as Health Protection Tools." *American Journal of Public Health,* 59:1613, September 1969. (Governmental responsibilities to establish and promote health protection standards.)

Hunt, E.: "Infant Mortality Trends and Maternal and Infant Care." *Children,* 17:88, May-June 1970.

Juberg, R. C.: "Heredity Counseling." *Nursing Outlook,* 14:28, January 1966. (Common counseling situations – abnormal children, childless marriage, known disease, premarital guidance, concern for next generation, racial ancestry, twins, biological father.)

Lang, D. M.: "Providing Maternity Care Through a Nurse-Midwifery Service Program." *Nursing Clinics of North America,* 4:509, September 1969. (Describes nurse-midwifery program and role of the nurse-midwife as a specialist.)

Lejeune, J.: "On the Nature of Men." *The American Journal of Human Genetics,* 22:121, March 1970. (Human genetics.)

Lubchenco, L. O.: "Assessment of Gestational Age and Development at Birth." *Pediatric Clinics of North America,* 17:125, February 1970. (Obstetric and pediatric clinical estimate; laboratory estimate; morbidity and mortality related to birth weight and gestational age.)

Mindlin, R., and Densen, P. M.: "Medical Care of Urban Infants: Continuity of Care." *American Journal of Public Health,* 59:1294, August 1969. (Correlations between such factors as socioeconomic status and ethnic background.)

Morris, R.: "The City of the Future and Planning for Health." *American Journal of Public Health,* 58:12, January 1968.

Nesbitt, R. E. L., and Richard, A. H.: "High-Risk Obstetrics." *American Journal of Obstetrics and Gynecology,* 103:972, April 1, 1969.

Peller, S.: "Proper Delineation of the Neonatal Period in Perinatal Mortality." *American Journal of Public Health,* 55:1005, July 1965. (Recommends limiting neonatal period to first postnatal week for determining mortality.)

Pittman, R.: "The Man in the Family." *Nursing Outlook,* 16:62, April 1968. (Cultural differences regarding role of man in family; nursing students' reactions to working with fathers.)

"Reducing Infant Mortality: Suggested Approaches." *Journal of the American Medical Association,* 193:310, July 26, 1965. (Mortality rates; definitions of rates; factors influencing mortality; high risk pregnancies; care needed.)

Rose, P. A.: "The High-Risk Mother-Infant Dyad – a Challenge for Nursing." *Nursing Forum,* VI:1:94, 1967.

Runnerstrom, L.: "Nurses' Approval, Attention Promotes Patients' Well-Being." *Hospital Topics,* 44:133, August 1966. (Concepts to consider; implications for nursing.)

Seacat, M., and Schlachter, L.: "Expanded Nursing Role in Prenatal and Infant Care." *American Journal of Nursing,* 68:222, April 1968. (Nurse's role in working with middle income, private patients and their obstetricians and pediatricians.)

Shapiro, S., and Abramowicz, M.: "Pregnancy Outcome Correlates Identified Through Medical Record-Based Information." *American Journal of Public Health,* 59:1629, September 1969. (Data related to the relationship between a broad variety of maternal conditions and pregnancy outcome.)

Slatin, M.: "Extra Protection for High-Risk Mothers and Babies." *American Journal of Nursing,* 67:1241, June 1967. (Study of a project in Nebraska; comprehensive preconception, prenatal, delivery and postnatal teaching for mothers with the focus on potential or actual high risk mothers.)

"United States Maternal Mortality." *Clinical Pediatrics,* 8:312, June 1969.

Wallace, H. M.: "Factors Associated with Perinatal Mortality and Morbidity." *Clinical Obstetrics and Gynecology,* 13:13, March 1970. (Trends in infant and neonatal mortality, with statistical data for the period 1920-1969; concept of high risk with criteria for inclusion.)

Watkins, E. L.: "Low-Income Negro Mothers – Their Decision to Seek Prenatal Care." *American Journal of Public Health,* 58:655, April 1968. (Emphasizes need for comprehensive maternity programs and concern for the individual.)

Wessel, M. A.: "Maternal and Child Nursing – as a Pediatrician Sees It." *Nursing Outlook,* 11:207, March 1963.

Wiedenbach, E.: "Family Nurse Practitioner for Maternal and Child Care." *Nursing Outlook,* 13:50, December 1965. (Focus should be on entire maternity cycle; role and qualifications of nurses.)

OTHER PUBLICATIONS

Health Services for Mothers and Children – Under Title V, Social Security Act. Washington, D.C., U.S. Department of Health, Education and Welfare, 1969.

Optimal Health Care for Mothers and Children, pp. 1-55. Washington, D.C., U.S. Department of Health, Education and Welfare, 1967. (Basic issues; components of care; planning; manpower.)

Ross Laboratories: "To Provide Optional Maternal and Infant Care." *Public Health Reports,* Vol. 10, Number 4, July-August 1970.

Ross Laboratories: *Can Maternity Nursing Meet Today's Challenge?* Columbus, Ohio, 1967. (Roundtable discussion: Nurse-midwifery, and concepts of maternity nursing.)

NOTES

Guide 3

THE WONDERS PLAN THEIR FAMILY

PART I. REVIEW OF ANATOMY AND PHYSIOLOGY

Amy Greene and Harold Wonder, engaged for nearly a year, are planning to be married shortly. They both want children, but not immediately after they marry. Twenty-one-year-old Amy has just graduated from college and is planning to teach elementary school after their marriage. Harold, 24 years of age, is just beginning his law practice in a small firm.

They have read several pamphlets about family planning but have many questions. Amy has come to her physician for guidance in selecting a contraceptive which will be acceptable to her and to Harold.

1. Before you can understand the process of conception, you must have knowledge of the anatomy and physiology of the male and female reproductive systems. How will you use this knowledge?

2. Refer to an anatomy and physiology textbook and review the male reproductive system. State the facts which are significant in terms of discussing family planning with childbearing families.

3. Refer to an anatomy and physiology textbook and review the female reproductive system. Identify the following structures on the diagram.

labia majora	vestibule	fallopian tubes
labia minora	hymen	uterus
mons veneris	bartholin glands	cervix
clitoris	ovaries	vagina
		perineum

4. The diagram on page 35 represents the menstrual cycle.

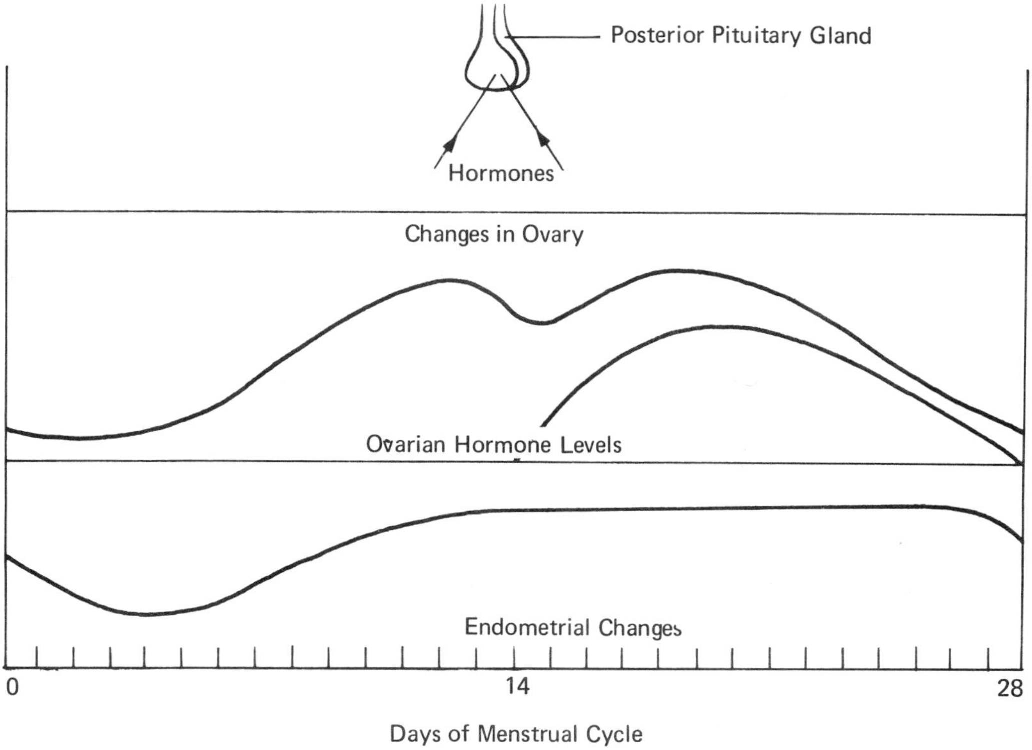

a. Identify the menstrual, proliferative and secretory phases of the menstrual cycle on the above diagram.

b. State how the endometrium changes during the:

1) Menstrual phase

2) Proliferative phase

3) Secretory phase

c. State the sequence of events which take place in the ovary during the menstrual cycle.

d. On the diagram line labeled "ovarian hormone levels," identify:

1) The sequence of events taking place during the menstrual cycle

2) When ovulation takes place

e. In the area labeled "ovarian hormone levels," identify the:

1) Estrogen hormone

2) Progesterone hormone

f. State the functions of:

1) Estrogen

2) Progesterone

g. Label the anterior pituitary gland on the diagram on page 34.

1) Identify the follicle-stimulating hormone and the leutinizing hormones secreted by the anterior pituitary gland.

2) State the functions of:

a) FSH (follicle-stimulating hormone)

b) LH (leutinizing hormone)

h. What is the function of the leutotropic hormone?

i. Which hormones are called gonadotropins?

5. a. When is it possible for conception to take place?

b. Show on the above diagram when conception could take place.

PART II. ASSISTING AMY WITH FAMILY PLANNING

6. Amy mentions she has seen several terms in her reading and asks you to clarify their meaning. State the meaning of the terms listed below.

a. Planned parenthood

b. Family planning

c. Birth planning

7. Amy would like some specific information about the various methods of contraception. For each of the methods listed on the chart on page 39, state its:

   a. Mechanism of action

   b. Advantages

   c. Disadvantages (include side effects and contraindications)

CONTRACEPTIVE METHOD	*MECHANISM OF ACTION*	*ADVANTAGES*	*DISADVANTAGES*
Coitus interruptus			
Condom			
Diaphragm			
Intrauterine device			
Oral contraceptive			
Rhythm			

CONTRACEPTIVE METHOD	*MECHANISM OF ACTION*	*ADVANTAGES*	*DISADVANTAGES*
Spermicidal preparation			

8. What factors will influence the method of contraception control selected by Amy and Harold?

PART III. STERILITY AND INFERTILITY IN CHILDBEARING COUPLES

Some couples seek guidance and medical evaluation because they are unable to conceive a child.

9. State the meaning of the terms sterility and infertility.

10. Why is it necessary for both husband and wife to be evaluated during the medical assessment of a childless couple?

11. State several of the factors predisposing to sterility and infertility.

12. State some of the measures used to diagnose sterility and infertility.

13. Select two problems of sterility and infertility and state how they might be managed medically.

14. What is the nurse's role in working with couples with impaired fertility?

15. What alternatives are available for the couple with impaired fertility who desire children?

REFERENCES

BOOKS

Anthony, E. J., and Benedek, T. (Ed.): *Parenthood – Its Psychology and Psychopathology.* Boston, Little Brown and Company, 1970.

Bergersen, B. S., and Krug, E. E.: *Pharmacology In Nursing.* 11th Ed. St. Louis, The C. V. Mosby Company, 1969.

Eastman, N. J., and Hellman, L. M.: *Williams Obstetrics.* 12th Ed., pp. 16-138. New York, Appleton-Century-Crofts, Inc., 1961.

Glass, R., and Kase, N.: *Woman's Choice.* New York, Basic Books, Inc., Publishers, 1970. (Guide to contraception, fertility, abortion and menopause.)

Guttmacher, A. F., et al.: *Planning Your Family.* New York, Macmillan Company, 1964.

Guyton, A. C.: *Textbook of Medical Physiology.* 3rd Ed., pp. 1035-1049, 1134-1169. Philadelphia, W. B. Saunders Company, 1966.

Hoffman, F., and Kleinman, R. (Eds.): *Advanced Concepts in Contraception.* Netherlands, Excerpta Medica Foundation, 1968.

Jacob, S. W., and Francone, C. A.: *Structure and Function in Man.* 2nd Ed. Philadelphia, W. B. Saunders Company, 1970.

Netter, F. H.: *The Ciba Collection of Medical Illustrations.* Volume 2: *Reproductive System.* New York, Ciba Corporation, 1964.

Rodman, M. J., and Smith, D. W.: *Pharmacology and Drug Therapy in Nursing.* Philadelphia, J. B. Lippincott Company, 1968.

Wiedenbach, E.: *Family-Centered Maternity Care.* 2nd Ed. New York, G. P. Putnam's Sons, 1967.

JOURNAL ARTICLES

Arnold, E.: "Individualizing Nursing Care in Family Planning." *Nursing Outlook,* 15:26, December 1967. (Knowledge and abilities needed by nurse.)

Behrman, S. J.: "Management of Infertility." *American Journal of Nursing,* 66:552, March 1966. (Evaluation and management of problems.)

Burks, J. L.: "Contraceptives for Students." *The Journal of Reproductive Medicine,* 4:9, February 1970.

Chesterman, H.: "The Public Health Nurse and Family Planning." *Nursing Outlook,* 12:32, September 1964. (Family planning as part of total MCH service; the nurse's feelings.)

Clark, T. H.: "Contraception When the Pill Isn't the Answer." *Patient Care,* III:94, May 1969.

Fischman, S. H.: "Choosing an Appropriate Contraceptive." *Nursing Outlook,* 15:28, December 1967. (Physiological basis of oral contraception, IUD, diaphragm, spermicides, vaginal suppositories and the rhythm method.)

Fredricsson, B., and Gullbring, B.: "A Study on the Influence of ABO Blood Groups on Fertility." *International Journal of Fertility,* 15:159, July-September 1970.

Gelber, I.: "Family Planning in a Growing World." *American Journal of Nursing,* 64:98, August 1964. (Overview of population growth and birth control; religion; contraceptives; planned parenthood; world population.)

Guttmacher, A. F.: "Family Planning, the Needs and the Methods." *American Journal of Nursing,* 69:1229, June 1969. (Historical and global aspects of family planning; current methods of contraception and abortion.)

Lane, M. E.: "Emotional Aspects of Contraception." *Bulletin of the American College of Nurse-Midwives,* XV:16, February 1970.

Luckey, E. B.: "Helping Children Grow Up Sexually – How? When? By Whom?" *Children,* 14:130, July-August 1967.

Manisoff, M. T.: "Counseling for Family Planning." *American Journal of Nursing,* 66:2671, December 1966.
Morgan, D. G.: "The Premarital Examination." *Clinical Obstetrics and Gynecology,* 6:539, September 1963.
Newton, M.: "Feminine Hygiene." *American Journal of Nursing,* 64:100, December 1964. (Hygiene of reproductive organs – reviews seven endocrine ages of girls and women.)
Pohlman, E., and Pohlman, J. M.: *The Psychology of Birth Planning.* Cambridge, Massachusetts, Schenkman Publishing Company, Inc., 1969. (The desire for children; costs of conception; husband-wife relationships; parental roles; unwanted conceptions and parents' feelings; methods of birth planning; psychological aspects of overpopulation.)
Schleisner, K. M.: "A Study of Intra-Uterine Contraceptive Devices." *American Journal of Nursing,* 66:2469, November 1966.
Semmens, J. P.: "Sex Education of the Prepubescent and Pubescent Female." *Clinical Obstetrics and Gynecology,* 11:757, September 1968.
Wall, R. L.: "Evaluation and Management of Infertility." *Clinical Obstetrics and Gynecology,* 12:851, December 1969.
Wallace, H. M., et al.: "Relationships Between Family Planning and Maternal and Child Health." *American Journal of Public Health,* 59:1355, August 1969.

OTHER PUBLICATIONS

Children's Bureau: *Family Planning.* Washington, D.C., U.S. Government Printing Office, U.S. Department of Health, Education and Welfare, 1966.
G. D. Searle and Company: *Family Planning with the Pill – a Manual for Nurses.* Chicago, 1968. (Population; family planning; anatomy and physiology; the pill; nurse's role in family planning.)
Ortho Pharmaceutical Corporation: *Understanding Conception and Contraception.* Raritan, New Jersey, 1968.
Swartz, D. P., and Vander Wiele, R. L.: *Methods of Conception Control.* Raritan, New Jersey, Ortho Pharmaceutical Corporation, 1967. (Programmed instruction; menstrual cycle; contraceptive methods.)

NOTES

Guide 4

THE WONDERS EXPECT THEIR FIRST BABY

On March 5th, Amy and Harold Wonder visit an obstetrician to confirm their belief that Amy is pregnant. The Wonders have been married for two years. Mr. Wonder, 26 years of age, is a lawyer in a small law firm; Mrs. Wonder, 23 years of age, has been employed as a third grade teacher for the past year. They live in a four-room apartment in a large city. They are here because Amy has missed two menstrual periods (her last period began January 10th), she feels nauseated nearly every day and she tires easily. Although they would like to have a baby very much, they had hoped to wait until the school year was over before Amy became pregnant.

"We had really planned on my being able to work this year . . . Except for being tired and sick to my stomach in the morning, I feel O.K. . . . We've always been very active and usually after work Harold and I will go bowling or play tennis or something. But now it's all I can do to go home, take a nap and fix supper!" Harold says to Amy: "I hope you are pregnant, honey. We can do without the extra money. You'll see." He turns to you and says, "So it'll be a little sooner than we had planned. It's O.K. I think it's great!"

1. Amy's and Harold's anticipation of the new baby is similar to that of some other expectant parents. What other reactions might expectant parents have on hearing they will be having a baby?

2. Amy is anxious to know when the baby will be due. Calculate the expected date of Amy's confinement (EDC). Her last menstrual period was January 10th.

3. Amy is to have a complete physical evaluation, including a pelvic examination.

   a. How will you prepare her, psychologically and physically, for the pelvic examination?

   b. What are the purposes of the pelvic measurements and vaginal examination?

4. a. What presumptive signs of pregnancy are evident from Amy's history?

   b. What presumptive signs are obtainable from Amy's physical and pelvic examination?

c. What presumptive sign cannot be noted at this initial visit of Amy's? When will it be evident?

5. What are the probable signs of pregnancy that Amy will exhibit? When can each of these signs first be noted?

6. What are the positive signs of pregnancy that Amy will exhibit? When will each of these signs first be noted?

7. Amy wants to know why she needs laboratory tests as part of her examination. State the reason for each of the laboratory tests listed below.

Blood: Wasserman

Group and type

Hemoglobin

Urine: Sugar

Albumin

Papanicolaou smear

8. Amy is said to be a primigravida, while her sister, who has had two children, is referred to by the obstetrician as a multipara. Define each of the following terms:

   a. Gravida

   b. Para

   c. Primigravida

   d. Multipara

9. There are several biological and chemical tests which could be performed to diagnose Amy's pregnancy. On the chart below:

   a. List at least three of these tests

   b. State the physiological basis for each of these tests

   c. State the information Mrs. Wonder would need if each of these tests were to be performed.

TEST	PHYSIOLOGICAL BASIS	INFORMATION

10. Throughout Amy's pregnancy, many anatomical and physiological changes will occur. As a result of these changes, Amy will experience various minor discomforts and complaints. For each of the following organs or systems, state the:

    a. Changes which occur

    b. Trimester in which the changes are expected to occur

    c. Physiological basis for each change

	CHANGES	WHEN OCCUR	BASIS
Uterus			
Cervix			

	CHANGES	*WHEN OCCUR*	*BASIS*
Vagina			
Breasts			
Skin			
Pelvis			
Abdominal wall			

	CHANGES	*WHEN OCCUR*	*BASIS*
Heart and circulatory system			
Respiratory system			
Digestive system			
Urinary system			

	CHANGES	*WHEN OCCUR*	*BASIS*
Basal metabolism			
Endocrine system			

11. As a result of these anatomical and physiological changes, Amy may experience various discomforts. Using the chart below, state:

    a. The discomforts Amy might have

    b. Suggestions you might give Amy to alleviate or manage each discomfort

    c. The scientific rationale for each of your suggestions

DISCOMFORT	*NURSE'S SUGGESTIONS*	*RATIONALE*

d. Mild nausea and vomiting are considered minor discomforts of pregnancy. If the condition persists and becomes severe, it is known as hyperemesis gravidarum, a major complication of pregnancy.

1) What is hyperemesis gravidarum?

2) How is hyperemesis gravidarum managed?

12. Assuming Mrs. Wonder has a normal pregnancy, how often will she probably be expected to visit the obstetrician during the:

a. First trimester

b. Second trimester

c. Third trimester

13. Amy states that she was surprised to find she had lost two pounds in the past two months because she thought she was supposed to gain weight when she was pregnant.

a. Explain the probable reasons for Amy's two-pound weight loss.

b. How much weight can Amy anticipate she may gain during her pregnancy?

c. What is the maximum she should gain each trimester? Why?

14. Amy will need some guidance in planning an adequate diet during her pregnancy.

a. What information do you need from Amy before you begin discussing her diet with her?

b. On the following chart, state:

1) Amy's average daily nutritional requirements before and during pregnancy in terms of the nutrients listed below.

2) Harold's daily requirements in relation to the nutrients below.

	AMY		*HAROLD*
	NONPREGNANT	*PREGNANT*	
Calories			
Protein			
Fat			

	AMY NONPREGNANT	AMY PREGNANT	HAROLD
Minerals			
Calcium			
Iron			
Vitamins			
A			
C			
D			
Thiamine			
Riboflavin			
Niacin			

c. How will these requirements influence Amy's meal planning?

d. What factors do you want to be certain Amy understands about her diet?

15. Amy is surprised when she hears that some pregnant women eat unusual substances, such as laundry starch. She asks you why this practice, known as pica, occurs.

a. What is pica?

b. What substances are commonly eaten by pregnant women?

c. What is the relationship between these substances and the mother's nutrition?

d. What implications does this have for nursing?

16. Mrs. Wonder has said she tires easily lately and needs a nap every afternoon.

    a. Why does Amy probably tire easily?

    b. Why is it important for Amy to receive sufficient rest and sleep?

    c. What knowledge do you need about Amy in order to help her plan to get this needed rest?

    d. What suggestions can you give the Wonders to help Amy get the rest she needs?

17. Mrs. Wonder wants to continue teaching until June and asks you if this would be advisable.

    a. What are your responsibilities in relation to this question?

    b. Briefly state the recommendations of the Children's Bureau for employment standards during childbearing.

18. Mrs. Wonder wants to know what type of clothing to purchase during her pregnancy if she "ever begins to gain any weight!"

    a. State the factors that need to be considered in advising her about clothing and shoes.

b. Compare the price Amy would pay for undergarments and outer garments in a chain store and in a maternity shop. Select two or three of each type of garment for comparison.

19. Amy needs to know what changes may occur during her pregnancy that would necessitate calling the physician immediately. On the chart below, state the:

a. Danger signals of which Amy needs to be aware

b. Significance of each danger signal

DANGER SIGNAL	*SIGNIFICANCE OF DANGER SIGNAL*

20. Amy seems overwhelmed with the information she has received and states: "My goodness, there is so much to remember! Is it all important? How can I ever remember all of this?"

    a. State how this feeling of being overwhelmed could be:

        1) Prevented

        2) Alleviated

    b. What factors need to be considered in determining how much to discuss with Amy (or any other pregnant woman) on her first visit to the obstetrician or clinic?

21. Three psychological tasks of the pregnant woman have been identified in the article, "Developmental Tasks of Pregnancy," by Leonide Tanner. List these three developmental tasks and for each task state:

    a. The trimester during which the task is being worked through

    b. Amy's expected behaviors as she is working through each of these tasks

c. The implications for nursing intervention

22. Amy is now seven months pregnant. Harold has come with her for her appointment. While Amy is seeing the obstetrician, Harold tells you he has noticed some changes in her behavior of which she seems unaware.

    a. What behavioral changes might Harold have noticed?

    b. What support can you offer Harold when Amy is experiencing these changes?

    c. What support can Harold give Amy?

23. During the seventh month of Amy's pregnancy, the Wonders question the advisability of taking a vacation to visit Harold's parents, 1200 miles away. What factors will the obstetrician consider in advising the Wonders about the trip?

24. Amy tells you of some of the advice and information she has received from relatives and friends. Some of this advice and information is commonly referred to as "old wives' tales." Cite at least two old wives' tales related to childbearing and state whether there is any validity in these tales.

25. Amy and Harold are likely to have fears and fantasies about the developing baby, whether these are expressed or not.

    a. What are the fears and fantasies frequently experienced by expectant parents?

    b. What is the nurse's role in helping the mother and father to cope with these fears and fantasies?

REFERENCES

BOOKS

Anthony, E. J., and Benedek, T. (Eds.): *Parenthood – Its Psychology and Psychopathology.* Boston, Little, Brown and Company, 1970.

Barnes, A. C.: "Prevention of Congenital Anomalies from the Point of View of the Obstetrician." *Congenital Malformations,* International Medical Congress, Limited, 1964. (Genetic counseling; prenatal care; maternal disease; pregnancy-related diseases; labor and delivery.)

Bing, E. D.: *Six Practical Lessons for an Easier Childbirth.* New York, Grosset and Dunlap, 1967.

Brandt, M. B.: "Nutrition in Pregnancy." In Lytle, N. A. (Ed.): *Maternal Health Nursing.* pp. 66-80. Iowa, William C. Brown Company, Inc., 1967.

Bryant, R. D., and Overland, A. E.: *Woodward and Gardner's Obstetric Management and Nursing,* 7th Ed. Philadelphia, F. A. Davis Company, 1964.

Buxton, C. L.: "Psychophysical Training in Preparation for Childbirth." In Lytle, N. A. (Ed.): *Maternal Health Nursing,* pp. 81-96. Iowa, William C. Brown Company, Inc., 1967. (Prenatal; labor.)

Buxton, C. L.: *A Study of Psychophysical Methods of Relief of Childbirth Pain.* Philadelphia, W. B. Saunders Company, 1962. (Natural childbirth; hypnosis; education.)

Chertok, L.: *Motherhood and Personality.* Philadelphia, J. B. Lippincott Company, 1969. (Includes psychosomatic methods of preparation for childbirth; case histories; critical review of literature on psychology of pregnancy, childbirth and preparation for childbirth.)

Dunston, Beverly N.: "Pica During Pregnancy." In Bergersen, B. S., et al. (Eds.): *Current Concepts in Clinical Nursing.* Vol. 2, pp. 268-279. St. Louis, The C. V. Mosby Company, 1969. (Includes extensive bibliography.)

Duvall, E. M.: *Family Development.* 3rd Ed., pp. 157-185. Philadelphia, J. B. Lippincott Company, 1971.

Eastman, N. J., and Hellman, L. M.: *Williams Obstetrics.* 12th Ed., pp. 221-279, 337-371. New York, Appleton-Century-Crofts, Inc., 1961.

Eastman, N. J., and Russell, K. P.: *Expectant Motherhood.* 5th Ed., revised. Boston, Little, Brown and Company, 1970.

Goodrich, F. W.: *Preparing for Childbirth: A Manual for Expectant Parents.* Englewood Cliffs, New Jersey, Prentice-Hall, 1966.

Grimm, R.: "Psychological and Social Factors in Pregnancy, Delivery, and Outcome." In Richardson, S. A., and Guttmacher, A. F. (Eds.): *Childbearing – Its Social and Psychological Aspects,* pp. 1-52. Baltimore, The Williams and Wilkins Company, 1967.

Illsley, R.: "The Sociological Study of Reproduction and Its Outcome." In Richardson, S. A., and Guttmacher, S. F. (Eds.): *Childbearing – Its Social and Psychological Aspects,* pp. 75-141. Baltimore, The Williams and Wilkins Company, 1967.

Jacob, S. W., and Francome, C. A.: *Structure and Function in Man,* 2nd Ed. Philadelphia, W. B. Saunders Company, 1970.

Lerch, C.: *Maternity Nursing.* St. Louis, The C. V. Mosby Company, 1970.

Montagu, A.: *Life Before Birth.* New York, New American Library, 1964. (Written for mothers; overview of fetal development, factors influencing fetal growth and development.)

Nesbitt, R. E. L.: "Primary Prevention from the Viewpoint of the Obstetrician." In Lytle, N. A. (Ed.): *Maternal Health Nursing,* pp. 31-49. Iowa, William C. Brown Company, Inc., 1967. (Prenatal care, prematurity, third trimester bleeding, fetal distress, toxemia, labor.)

Netter, F. H.: *The Ciba Collection of Medical Illustrations.* Vol. 2. *Reproductive System.* New York, Ciba Corporation, 1965.

Nordmark, M. T., and Rohweder, A. W.: *Scientific Foundations of Nursing.* 2nd Ed., pp. 323-329. Philadelphia, J. B. Lippincott Company, 1967.

Schaefer, G., and Zisowitz, M. L.: *The Expectant Father.* New York, Simon and Schuster, 1964.

Tanner, L. M.: "Developmental Tasks of Pregnancy." In Bergersen, B. S., et al. (Eds.): *Current Concepts in Clinical Nursing.* Vol. 2, Chapter 28. St. Louis, The C. V. Mosby Company, 1969.

Williams, S. R.: *Nutrition and Diet Therapy.* St. Louis, The C. V. Mosby Company, 1969.

Ziegel, E., and Van Blarcom, C. C.: *Obstetric Nursing.* 5th Ed., pp. 89-148. New York, The Macmillan Company, 1965.

JOURNAL ARTICLES

Auerbach, A. B.: "Meeting the Needs of New Mothers." *Children,* 11:223, November-December 1964. (Psychological and social needs of new and expectant parents; implications for care.)

Buchsbaum, S. J.: "Accidental Injury Complicating Pregnancy." *American Journal of Obstetrics and Gynecology,* 102:752, November 1, 1968.

Clark, A. L.: "The Beginning Family." *American Journal of Nursing,* 66:802, April 1966. (The phases of establishment, childbearing and childrearing; postpartal needs; teaching.)

Dwyer, J. T., et al.: "Management of Weight in Pregnancy." *Postgraduate Medicine,* 48:208, July 1970. (Goals of weight gain; pattern of gain; preconception management in obese and in underweight women.)

"14 Institutions Keep Track of 60,000 Infants: Poorly Nourished Mothers Major Birth Defect Focus." *JAMA Medical News,* 204:24, May 20, 1968.

Fugo, N. W.: "Management of Common Problems of Prenatal Care." *Clinical Obstetrics and Gynecology,* 6:627, September 1963.

Glynn, E. M.: "Nursing Support During Intra-Uterine Transfusions." *American Journal of Nursing,* 65:72, August 1965.

Gold, E. M.: "Interconceptional Nutrition." *Journal of the American Dietetic Association,* 55:27, July 1969. (Emphasizes nutritional status of teenagers and underweight and overweight patients when not pregnant as necessary for healthier babies.)

Hendrick, W.: "An Elderly Primigravida Takes a 'Refresher Course' in Obstetrics." *American Journal of Nursing,* 70:787, April 1970. (Compares her pregnancy with textbook picture; describes care received; states that the care not received was appalling.)

Larsen, V. L.: "Stresses of the Childbearing Year." *American Journal of Public Health,* 56:32, January 1966. (Stresses during pregnancy, labor and delivery; postpartum and first three months at home.)

Lorincz, A. B.: "The Initial Examination of the Prenatal Patient." *Clinical Obstetrics and Gynecology,* 6:562, September 1963.

McCain, F. R.: "Nursing by Assessment – Not Intuition." *American Journal of Nursing,* 65:82, April 1965.

Moore, M. L.: "The Clay Eaters." *RN,* 33:44, August 1970. (Pica during pregnancy.)

"The Mother's Changing Needs." *Briefs,* 32:79, May 1968.

Newton, N.: "Emotions of Pregnancy." *Clinical Obstetrics and Gynecology,* 6:639, September 1963 (and *Child and Family,* 4:3, Summer 1965). (Reactions to pregnancy; fears, worries, food cravings, mood changes; psychosomatic disorders; abortion; effect of woman's emotions on the family.)

"The Prenatal Visit." *Clinical Pediatrics,* 9:309, May 1970. (A letter from pediatrician to prospective parents recommending prenatal visit to prediatrician. Comments pro and con these visits.)

Rubin, R.: "Cognitive Style in Pregnancy." *American Journal of Nursing,* 70:502, March 1970. (Changes in pregnancy; period of inconclusive questioning and uncertainty.)

Sailor, N. M.: "Nutrition Knowledge Applied to Everyday Living." *Nursing Outlook,* 9:756, December 1961. (Significance of food to individuals; the basic four; suggestions for teaching.)

Schaefer, G.: "The Expectant Father." *Nursing Outlook,* 14:46, September 1966. (Feelings and behaviors of expectant fathers; suggests ways husband can help wife.)

Shank, R. E.: "A Chink in Our Armour." *Nutrition Today,* 5:2, Summer 1970. (Guidelines for new approach to dietary management of pregnancy, including adolescents, anemia, toxemia.)

Sundberg, A. M.: "Influencing Prenatal Behavior." *American Journal of Public Health,* 56:1218, August 1966. (Comprehensive maternity care program in Baltimore; role of nursing, social service, dental service, nutrition service and health education.)

Wessel, M. A.: "Maternal and Child Nursing – as a Pediatrician Sees It." *Nursing Outlook,* 11:207, March 1963.

Williams, B.: "Sleep Needs During the Maternity Cycle." *Nursing Outlook,* 15:53, February 1967.

Vander Zanden, J. W., and Vander Zanden, M. V.: "The Interview." *Nursing Outlook,* 11:743, October 1963. (What questions to ask and how.)

OTHER PUBLICATIONS

Auerbach, A. B., and Arnstein, H. S.: *Pregnancy and You.* Child Study Association, 1962.

Carnation Company: *Pregnancy in Anatomical Illustrations.* 1969.

Children's Bureau: *Eat Well for You and Your Baby Who Is on the Way.* Washington, D.C., U.S. Government Printing Office, U.S. Department of Health, Education and Welfare, 1969.

Children's Bureau: *Prenatal Care.* Washington, D.C., U.S. Government Printing Office, U.S. Department of Health, Education and Welfare, 1962.

Children's Bureau: *When Your Baby is On the Way.* Washington, D.C., U.S. Government Printing Office, U.S. Department of Health, Education and Welfare, 1961.

Highly, B. L.: "Antepartal Nursing Intervention." *Conference on Maternal and Child Nursing Current Concepts in Nursing Care.* Columbus, Ohio, Ross Laboratories, 1964.

Runnerstrom, L.: "Food Iron Intake and Hemoglobin Levels in Uncomplicated Pregnancy: Implications for Nursing." *Clinical Sessions,* Number 11, pp. 28-30, New York, American Nurses Association, 1964.

NOTES

Guide 5

BABY WONDER'S DEVELOPMENT

Amy and Harold Wonder are expecting their first baby. During the 10 lunar months of Amy's pregnancy, Baby Wonder will grow from a single cell to an infant weighing approximately 7 pounds. An understanding of how this development takes place is essential to providing optimal nursing care for this family.

1. How will an understanding of Baby Wonder's development be useful in providing nursing care?

2. Amy has a 28-day menstrual cycle; thus conception took place approximately________days prior to the onset of her next menstrual period.

3. Why are lunar months used when referring to Baby Wonder's development?

4. On the diagram below:

   a. Label the following structures:

ovary	external os
fallopian tube	internal os
fundus	endometrium
uterine cavity	myometrium
cervix	perimetrium
vagina	

b. Trace the path of the ovum from the ovary until it is fertilized by the sperm.

c. Trace the path of the sperm from the vagina until it fertilizes the ovum.

d. Trace the path of the fertilized ovum to the implantation site.

e. Draw and label the three layers of the decidua.

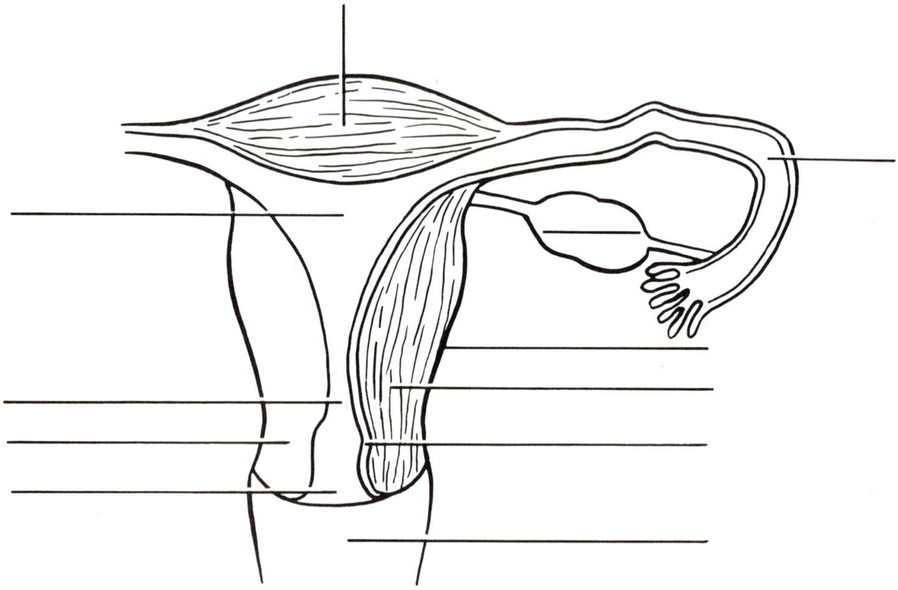

5. a. What is the decidua?

b. What happens to the decidua after the birth of the baby?

6. Approximately how many days does it take for the fertilized ovum to become implanted in the uterus?

7. State the hormonal adaptation of Mrs. Wonder's body which promotes her adjustment to the demands of pregnancy and suppresses menstruation.

8. Using the following schematic representation as a guide:

   a. Briefly describe the changes which occur in the fertilized ovum.

   b. Define any terms with which you are unfamiliar.

   (additional space for definitions on page 74)

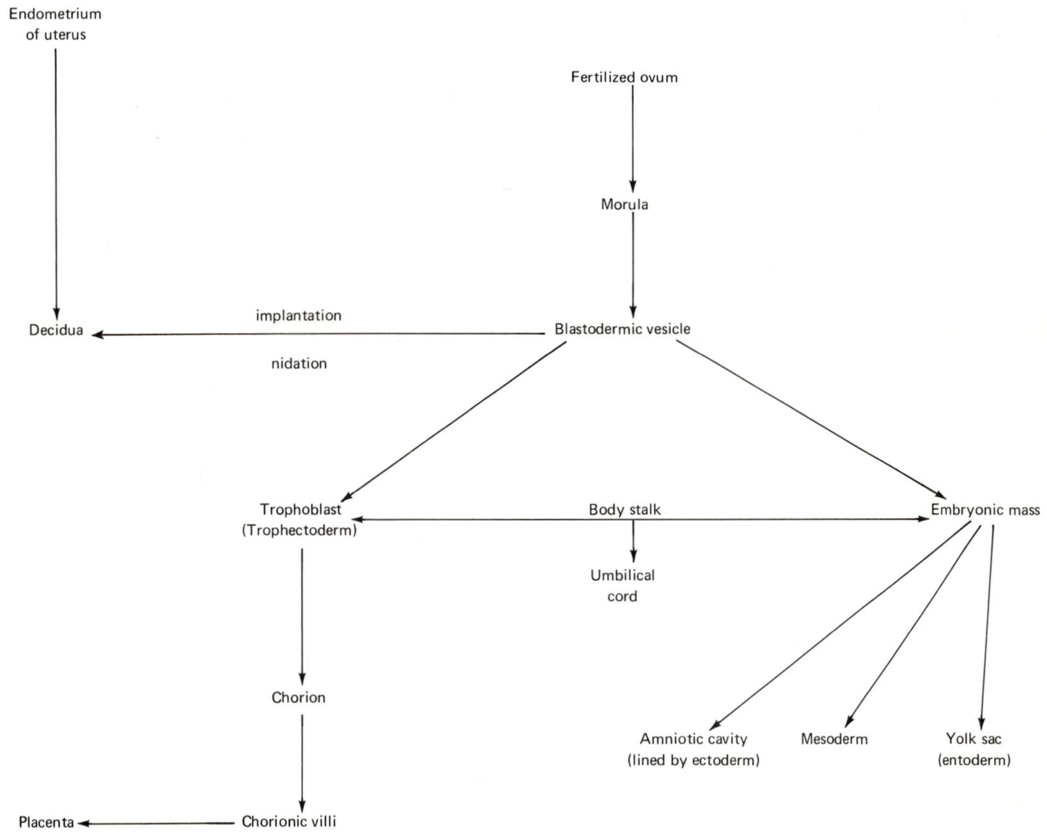

9. The cells of the morula become differentiated into three layers. State the fetal structures which will arise from the ectoderm, the mesoderm and the entoderm.

10. a. When does development of the placenta occur?

    b. What are the functions of the placenta?

c. Describe the maternal and fetal sides of the placenta.

d. What is meant by the placental barrier?

e. What effect does the placental barrier have on the transfer of substances between the placenta and the fetus?

11. How is the embryo nourished prior to development of the placenta?

12. Describe the following conditions and state how each would affect the development of the fetus.

    a. Poorly implanted placenta

b. Placenta previa

c. Abruptio placenta

d. Ectopic pregnancy

13. What changes take place in the placenta when a pregnancy goes beyond 40 weeks? How does this affect the fetus?

14. a. State the environmental factors which will influence Baby Wonder's development in utero.

b. How will knowledge of these factors influence anticipatory guidance of the Wonders?

15. Baby Wonder's heredity is dependent upon the chromosomes and genes received from his parents.

    a. Differentiate between the following terms:

        1) Chromosomes and genes

        2) Meiosis and mitosis

        3) Autosomes and sex chromosomes

        4) Homozygous and heterozygous

        5) Spermatogenesis and oogenesis

    b. How many chromosomes will Baby Wonder have?

    c. Is Baby Wonder's sex determined by his mother's or his father's sex chromosomes?

    d. Baby Wonder's chromosomes can be studied by karyotyping. What does karyotype mean?

e. Fetal malformations may be caused by modifications of genetic or chromosomal structure. Give several examples of:

1) Genetic abnormalities

2) Chromosomal abnormalities

f. What implications do these genetic and chromosomal abnormalities have for genetic counseling?

16. Amy says identical twins run in Harold's family. What is the difference between identical and fraternal twins?

17. Amy has heard that many things can happen to the baby or to the mother which will affect the baby's development. She questions you about several of these. State the specific scientific facts you need in order to answer these questions.

a. "What happens if I get rubella while I'm pregnant? Can I get the rubella vaccine?"

b. "I've heard that x-rays are bad while you are pregnant, and even before. Is this true?"

c. "Is it true that if I take any drugs during pregnancy they will hurt the baby? I'm sure I took aspirin before I knew I was pregnant."

d. "Does smoking really have a bad effect on the baby?"

e. "I know someone who is 37 and is having a baby. She's afraid the baby will be retarded. Will it?"

18. You will find the terms embryo and fetus used in referring to Baby Wonder's development. Differentiate between these two terms.

19. Baby Wonder is surrounded by amniotic fluid.

    a. What is amniotic fluid? How is it formed? What are its functions?

    b. What would be the significance of polyhydramnios to:

        1) Baby Wonder?

        2) Amy Wonder?

20. Baby Wonder's appearance and characteristics change rapidly while he is in utero. For each of the designated times on the following chart:

    a. State the embryonic or fetal:

        1) Length

        2) Weight

        3) At least two to four anatomical or physiological developmental characteristics

    b. When appropriate, state the changes in Amy that are directly related to the development of Baby Wonder which can be noted by Amy or her obstetrician.

AGE	*LENGTH*	*WEIGHT*	*BABY WONDER'S CHARACTERISTIC*	*CHANGES IN AMY*
4 weeks				
8 weeks				
12 weeks				
16 weeks				

AGE	LENGTH	WEIGHT	BABY WONDER'S CHARACTERISTIC	CHANGES IN AMY
20 weeks				
24 weeks				
32 weeks				
36 weeks				

21. Stated below are some of the characteristics of human growth and development which are applicable to Baby Wonder's embryonic and fetal development.

    a. Explain, in your own words, what is meant by each statement.

    b. Give an example to demonstrate each characteristic. Refer to your answer to Question 20 and to Figure 1 for examples.

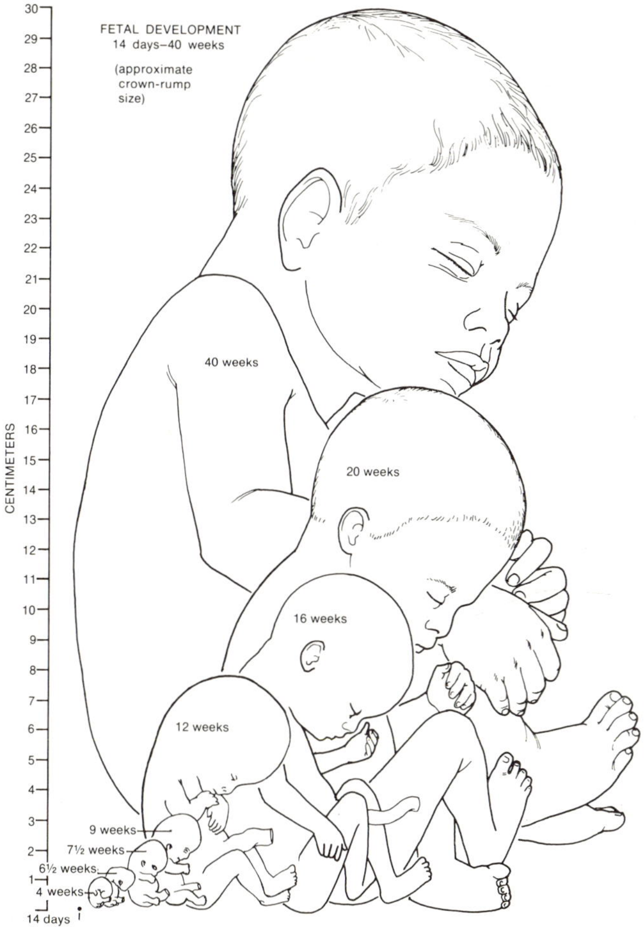

(Illustration adapted from Arey: *Developmental Anatomy* 7th Ed., Philadelphia, W. B. Saunders Co., 1965, p. 101.
Fitzpatrick et al.: *Maternity Nursing,* 11th Ed. Philadelphia, J. B. Lippincott Co., 1966, pp. 82 and 83.
Understanding Conception and Contraception. Raritan, N. J., Ortho Pharmaceutical Corporation, 1968, pp. 41-45).

1) Development follows a regular pattern.

2) Development is continuous.

3) Development proceeds from general to specific responses.

4) Development occurs at different rates for different parts of the body.

5) Development is predictable.

22. Label the following structures on the diagram of the fetal skull:

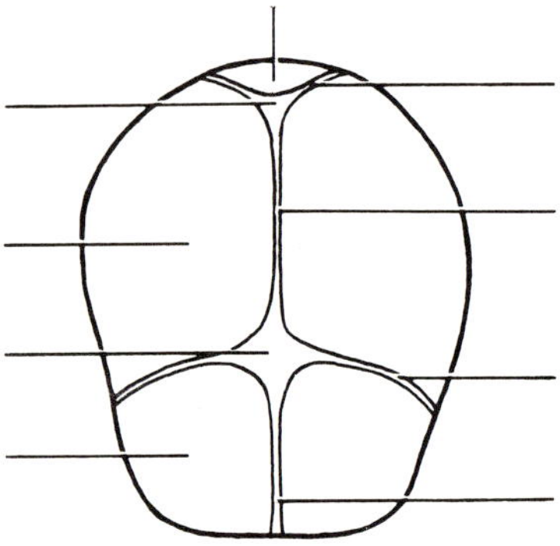

FETAL SKULL

parietal bone
frontal bone
occiput
sagittal suture
lambdoid suture
coronal suture
frontal suture
anterior fontanel
posterior fontanel

23. The schematic diagram below represents Baby Wonder's fetal circulation.

FETAL CIRCULATION

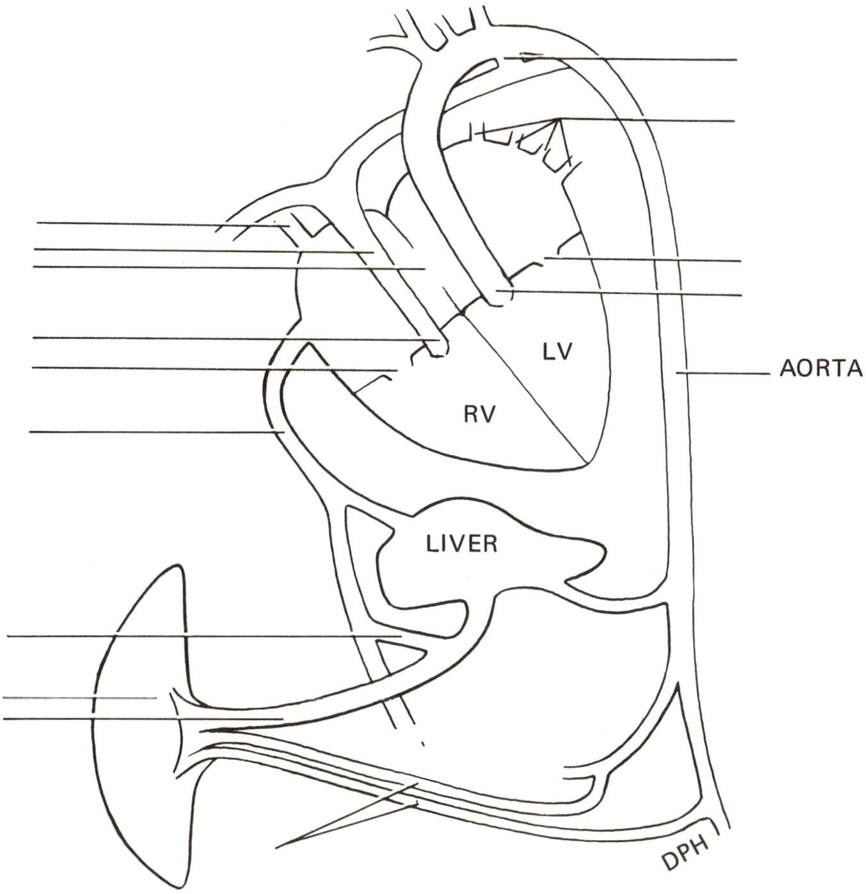

a. Label the following structures:

right atrium	left atrium
pulmonary artery	mitral valve
tricuspid valve	aortic valve
pulmonic valve	superior vena cava
inferior vena cava	pulmonary veins
foramen ovale	placenta
ductus arteriosus	umbilical arteries
ductus venosus	umbilical vein

b. Using the diagram on page 85, trace the circulation of the blood from the placenta through the fetus and returning to the placenta.

c. State the function in the fetus of the following structures:

1) ductus arteriosus

2) foramen ovale

3) ductus venosus

4) umbilical vein

5) umbilical arteries

6) liver

24. Evidence indicative of fetal distress must receive prompt attention if Baby Wonder is to be wellborn.

    a. What is fetal distress?

    b. State the signs and symptoms indicative of possible fetal distress which might be displayed by:

        1) Amy

        2) Baby Wonder

    c. What methods are available to obstetricians for anticipating or determining fetal distress?

    d. What is the nurse's role when fetal distress is anticipated or present?

25. Considerable emphasis is now being placed on medical care of the fetus in order to increase the chances of all babies being wellborn. How do these trends in fetal care affect the role of the nurse?

26. How can your knowledge of Baby Wonder's fetal development be utilized while working with the Wonders?

REFERENCES

BOOKS

Adamsons, K. (Ed.): *Diagnosis and Treatment of Fetal Disorders.* New York, Springer-Verlag New York, Inc., 1968.

Arey, L. B.: *Developmental Anatomy.* 7th Ed. Philadelphia, W. B. Saunders Company, 1965.

Eastman, N. J., and Hellman, L. M.: *Williams Obstetrics.* 12th Ed., pp. 140-217. New York, Appleton-Century-Crofts, Inc., 1961.

Eastman, N. J., and Russell, K. P.: *Expectant Motherhood.* 5th Ed., revised. Boston, Little, Brown and Company, 1970. (Pregnancy; labor and delivery; postpartum; fetal development; newborn.)

Fishbein, M. (Ed.): *Birth Defects.* Philadelphia, J. B. Lippincott Company, 1963. (Genetics; fetal development; chromosomal and other defects; cause, prevention, treatment of defects; effect on child, family, society.)

Fitzpatrick, E., et al.: *Maternity Nursing.* 11th Ed. Philadelphia, J. B. Lippincott Company, 1966.

Flanagan, G. L.: *The First Nine Months of Life.* New York, Simon and Schuster, 1962. (Fetal development in pictures and narration.)

Gilbert, M. S.: *Biography of the Unborn.* New York, Hafner Publishing Company, 1963. (Nontechnical description of fetal development written for the layman; illustrated.)

Gruenberg, E. M.: "On the Psychosomatics of the Not-So-Perfect Fetal Parasite." In Richardson, S. A., and Guttmacher, A. F. (Eds.): *Childbearing – Its Social and Psychological Aspects,* pp. 53-74. Baltimore, The Williams and Wilkins Company, 1967.

Guyton, A. C.: *Textbook of Medical Physiology.* 3rd Ed., pp. 1170-1182. Philadelphia, W. B. Saunders Company, 1966.

Hasselmeyer, E. G.: "Indices of Fetal Welfare." In Bergersen, B. S., et al. (Eds.): *Current Concepts in Clinical Nursing.* Vol. 2, pp. 289-317. St. Louis, The C. V. Mosby Company, 1969. (Science of fetology and major areas of emphasis; biophysical, biochemical, and behavioral considerations of fetal welfare.)

Huntingford, P. J., Huter, K. A., and Saling, E. (Eds.): *Perinatal Medicine.* New York, Academic Press, 1969. (Amniotic fluid analysis; Rh incompatibility; electronic fetal heart monitoring; fetal blood sampling; clinical relationships between mother and fetus during labor; resuscitation of newborn, high-risk baby; diagnosis of respiratory disturbances in newborn.)

Kormondy, E. J.: *Introduction to Genetics: A Program for Self-Instruction.* New York, McGraw-Hill Book Company, 1964.

Montagu, A.: *Life Before Birth.* New York, New American Library, 1964. (Written for mothers; overview of fetal development, factors influencing fetal growth and development.)

Nesbitt, R. E. L.: "Primary Prevention from the Viewpoint of the Obstetrician." In Lytle, N. A.: *Maternal Health Nursing,* pp. 31-49. Iowa, William C. Brown Company, Inc., 1967. (Prenatal care; prematurity; third trimester bleeding; fetal distress; toxemia; labor.)

Netter, F. H.: *The Ciba Collection of Medical Illustrations.* Vol. 2. *Reproductive System.* New York, Ciba Corporation, 1965.

Stone, L. J., and Church, J.: *Childhood and Adolescence* 2nd Ed. New York, Random House, 1968.

Thompson, J. S., and Thompson, M. W.: *Genetics in Medicine,* pp. 4-16, 253-265. Philadelphia, W. B. Saunders Company, 1966. (Basis of heredity, including chromosomes, mitosis, meiosis, spermatogenesis and oogenesis; application to medical practice and public health.)

Whipple, D. V.: *Dynamics of Development: Euthenic Pediatrics,* pp. 18-29. New York, McGraw-Hill Book Company, 1966. (Mortality rates; causes.)

Williams, P. L., Wendell-Smith, C. P., and Treadgold, S.: *Basic Human Embryology.* Philadelphia, J. B. Lippincott Company, 1966.

Ziegel, E. and Van Blarcom, C. C.: *Obstetric Nursing.* 5th Ed., pp. 45-85. New York, The Macmillan Company, 1965.

JOURNAL ARTICLES

Adams, F. H.: "Functional Development of the Fetal Lung." *Journal of Pediatrics,* 68:794, May 1966. (Respiration-like movements in utero; contents of respiratory tract; blood flow and metabolism in lung; possible clinical implications.)

"Amnion: Protector of the Unborn Baby." *Briefs,* 32:131, November 1968. (Functions of amniotic fluid; protection, support [weightlessness], stability of environment [temperature], and aid in labor [composition of fluid].)

Amoroso, E. C.: "Development of the Early Embryo." *Science Journal,* 6:58, June 1970. (Description and illustrations of embryonic development.)

Apgar, V.: "Drugs in Pregnancy." *American Journal of Nursing,* 65:104, March 1965. (Reviews previous studies; lists medications and effect on fetus or neonate.)

Apgar, V., and Stickle, G.: "Birth Defects." *Journal of the American Medical Association,* 204:371, April 29, 1968. (Definition and taxonomy; fetal loss; prevalence.)

Bellam, G.: "The First Year of Life." *American Journal of Nursing,* 69:1244, June 1969. (Reviews fetal development; characteristics of newborn; some development through 12 months.)

Bishop, E. H.: "Ultrasonic Fetal Monitoring." *Clinical Obstetrics and Gynecology,* 11:1154, December 1968. (Ausculatory monitoring – advantages and disadvantages; use of ultrasonic monitoring.)

Buncher, C. R.: "Cigarette Smoking and Duration of Pregnancy." *American Journal of Obstetrics and Gynecology,* 103:942, April 1969. (Effects of smoking on gestation.)

Carbary, L. J.: "The Fetal Heart Monitor." *Nursing Outlook,* 11:835, November 1963. (Describes use of monitor by nurse.)

Cromb, E.: "The Diagnostic Use of Ultrasound in Obstetrics." *Bulletin of the American College of Nurse-Midwives,* XV:8, February 1970.

Douglas, G. W.: "Rubella in Pregnancy." *American Journal of Nursing,* 66:2664, December 1966.

"Drug Hazards to the Premature." *JAMA Medical News,* 203:26, January 29, 1968. (Physiological immaturity; effect of drugs by mother during pregnancy and labor.)

"Fetal Reaction to and Survival After Labor and Birth." *Child and Family,* 4:4, Fall 1965. (Intrauterine environment; effect of labor on infant; abnormal pregnancy and labor; normal newborn, complications of newborn period.)

Freda, V. J., and Robertson, J. G.: "Amniotic Fluid Analysis in Rh Iso-Immunization." *American Journal of Nursing,* 65:64, August 1965. (Detailed description of amniocentesis; how results of fluid analysis are used; several case illustrations.)

Goldstein, H., et al.: "Cigarette Smoking and Prematurity." *Public Health Reports,* 79:553, July 1964.

Hardy, J. B., and Gilkeson, M. R.: "Adverse Fetal Outcome Following Maternal Rubella after the First Trimester of Pregnancy." *Journal of the American Medical Association,* 207:2414, March 31, 1969. (Effects on infants when maternal rubella occurs between 14th and 31st weeks of pregnancy.)

Horstmann, D. M.: "Rubella and the Rubella Syndrome, Problems and Progress." *Medical Clinics of North America,* 51:587, May 1967. (Epidemiology, intrauterine rubella and rubella syndrome; problems of rubella in pregnancy.)

Hughs, E. C.: "Life in Inner Space." *American Journal of Nursing,* 63:92 January 1963.

James, L. S., et al.: "Respiratory Physiology of the Fetus and Newborn Infant." *New England Journal of Medicine,* 271:1403, December 31, 1964.

Katz, R. G., et al.: "Maternal and Congenital Rubella." *Clinical Pediatrics,* 7:323, June 1968. (Acquired and congenital rubella; incidence, clinical and laboratory findings, management.)

Kendall, B., and Farell, D. M.: "Uses of Fetal Electrocardiography." *American Journal of Nursing,* 64:75, July 1964. (How FECG is obtained; its uses.)

Larsen, G. L.: "What Every Nurse Should Know about Congenital Syphilis." *Nursing Outlook,* 13:52, March 1965. (Facts about syphilis; nursing implications.)

Little, W. A.: "Drugs in Pregnancy." *American Journal of Nursing,* 66:1303, June 1966.

McKay, R. J., and Lucey, J. F.: "Neonatalogy." *The New England Journal of Medicine,* 270:1231, June 4, 1964. (Drugs; immunity; respiratory distress syndrome; infants of diabetic mothers; hypoglycemia.)

McKay, R. J., and Lucey, J. F.: "Neonatology." *The New England Journal of Medicine,* 270:1292, June 11, 1964. (Jaundice; twins; prematurity; aids to diagnosing neonatal disease.)

Matousek, I.: "Fetal Nursing During Labor." *Nursing Clinics of North America,* 3:307, June 1968. (Proposed routine for fetal nursing; importance of mother and fetal assessment and care.)

Mulcahy, R., and Knaggs, J. F.: "Effect of Age, Parity, and Cigarette Smoking on Outcome of Pregnancy." *American Journal of Obstetrics and Gynecology,* 101:844, July 15, 1968.
"The New Rubella Virus Vaccine." *Clinical Pediatrics,* 8:410, July 1969. (Live vaccine; recommendations for use; precautions.)
Prystowsky, H.: "Intrauterine Growth and Development of the Baby." *Clinical Obstetrics and Gynecology,* 6:544, September 1963. (Fetal respiration; circulation; metabolic processes; neonatal blood counts; some abnormal neonatal conditions.)
Raventos, A.: "Weighing the Risk of Fetal Damage – X-Rays in Pregnancy." *American Journal of Nursing,* 66:1308, June 1966. (Hazards and risks to fetus and embryo of x-rays, recommendations regarding use.)
Smith, D. I.: "The Nurse's Role in Fetal Medicine." *Nursing Clinics of North America,* 1:121, March 1966. (Role regarding hazards to fetus and fetal transfusion.)
Sutherland, J. M., and Light, I. J.: "The Effect of Drugs upon the Developing Fetus." *Pediatric Clinics of North America,* 12:781, August 1965. (Includes many specific drugs.)

OTHER PUBLICATIONS

Abbott Laboratories: *The Human Placenta.* North Chicago, Spring 1956.
Carnation Company: *Pregnancy in Anatomical Illustrations.* 1969.
Ortho Pharmaceutical Corporation: *Understanding Conception and Contraception.* Raritan, New Jersey, 1968.

NOTES

Guide 6

PLANNING EXPECTANT PARENT EDUCATION

Amy and Harold Wonder would like to attend education classes for expectant parents. The Wonders are a young couple expecting their first baby. Amy says they do not know what to expect from these classes nor how to find out what classes are available in their community.

1. How can the nurse and Mrs. Wonder determine what types of parent education classes are offered in her community?

2. State the types of expectant parent classes available in:

   a. Your community

   b. The nation

3. What are the advantages and limitations of the Wonders' attending expectant parent classes?

4. Once the Wonders know the type of classes available to them, what factors will influence the class they select?

5. Mrs. Wonder would like to know why it is said that preparation for parenthood begins early in the parents' infancy.

   a. What aspects of an individual's infancy and childhood are thought to be influential in determining his or her characteristics as a parent?

b. Briefly state how and where preparation for parenthood is acquired throughout childhood.

6. Mrs. Wonder asks if all the terms she has seen in her reading related to education for childbearing and childrearing mean the same thing. These terms include parent education, education for childbirth, expectant parent education, prenatal education and education for family living. State the meaning of these various terms used in the literature so you can clarify them for Mrs. Wonder.

7. The Wonders need "anticipatory guidance" during their childbearing and childrearing years.

   a. What is "anticipatory guidance"?

   b. What are the advantages of anticipatory guidance for the Wonders?

You will be planning a series of classes for expectant parents. Listed below are some considerations to be made prior to beginning the classes.

8. State the factors to be considered in determining:

   a. Whether parent education should be on an individual or group basis

   b. If the class should be for expectant mothers, for expectant fathers, or for both parents

c. Whether the class should be for married and unmarried mothers together or separately

d. Who should do the teaching for the classes (such as lay groups, nurses, physicians)

e. How many classes will be in a series and how frequently the classes should meet

f. The content for a series of classes

g. Whether classes should be a formal presentation of content or group discussion

9. a. What is generally covered in the conventional preparation for parents' classes?

b. State any changes that you believe should be made in this content (such as additions or deletions) and the reasons for these changes.

10. Natural childbirth and psychoprophylactic childbirth (Lamaze method) necessitate the attendance of expectant parents at classes.

    a. State the similarities and differences between natural childbirth and psychoprophylactic childbirth.

    b. What specific preparation does the mother need if she selects one of these methods for childbirth?

11. a. What visual aids (such as types of films, charts, equipment) are available for teaching expectant parents?

b. State the factors which will determine:

1) Whether you will use these materials

2) How they will be used

12. Select one pamphlet or booklet which is available for expectant parents.

a. Name the pamphlet you have selected.

b. State the general criteria you need to consider in determining whether this pamphlet would be appropriate for Mrs. Wonder (such as accuracy of content).

c. Using the criteria listed above, evaluate this pamphlet in terms of its appropriateness for use by Mrs. Wonder.

13. State the principles of the teaching-learning process you should be able to use if you are going to teach expectant parent classes.

14. a. State how people's different social, economic and cultural situations will influence your planning of expectant parents' classes.

b. Select one socioeconomic level and one cultural group other than your own and give an example of adaptation in teaching that would be necessitated by that specific:

1) Socioeconomic group

2) Cultural group

15. a. Select a specific expectant parents' class you plan to teach.

b. State at least three objectives for the class you are planning.

c. Select one of these objectives and state how you would attempt to meet this objective.

d. State how you would evaluate whether the objective you have selected had been met.

REFERENCES

BOOKS

Auerbach, A. B.: *Parents Learn Through Discussion: Principles and Practices of Parent Group Education,* pp. 21-28, 40-54, 126-140, 180-190. New York, John Wiley and Sons, Inc., 1968.

Bing, E. D.: *Six Practical Lessons for an Easier Childbirth.* New York, Grosset and Dunlap, 1967.

Bing, E. D. (Ed.): *The Adventure of Birth.* New York, Simon and Schuster, 1970. (Accounts by mothers and fathers of their experience with the Lamaze method of childbirth.)

Bookmiller, M. M., et al.: *Textbook of Obstetrics and Obstetric Nursing.* 5th Ed. Philadelphia, W. B. Saunders Company, 1967.

Brim, O. G., Jr.: *Education for Child Rearing,* pp. 17-27. New York, The Free Press, 1965. (Definitions and objectives of parent education.)

Buxton, C. L.: *A Study of Psychophysical Methods of Relief of Childbirth Pain.* Philadelphia, W. B. Saunders Company, 1962. (Natural childbirth; hypnosis; education.)

Chabon, I.: *Awake and Aware: Participating in Childbirth Through Prophylaxis.* New York, Delacorte Press, 1966. (Paperback, New York, Dell Publishing Company, Inc. 1969.)

Clark, A. L.: *Leadership Technique in Expectant Parent Education.* New York, Springer Publishing Company, Inc. 1962.

Corbin, H.: In Goldston, I.: *The Family: A Focal Point in Health Education,* pp. 92-105. New York, International Universities Press, Inc., 1961. (Education for parenthood.)

Davis, M. E., and Rubin, R.: *DeLee's Obstetrics for Nurses.* 18th Ed., pp. 481-491. Philadelphia, W. B. Saunders Company, 1966. (Classes for expectant parents.)

Eastman, N. J., and Russell, K. P.: *Expectant Motherhood.* 5th Ed., revised. Boston, Little, Brown and Company, 1970. (Pregnancy; labor and delivery; postpartum; fetal development; newborn.)

Fitzpatrick, E., Eastman, N. J., and Reeder, R. S.: *Maternity Nursing.* 11th Ed., pp. 170-184. Philadelphia, J. B. Lippincott Company, 1966. (Parents' classes; education for natural and psychoprophylactic childbirth.)

Goodrich, F. W.: *Preparing for Childbirth: A Manual for Expectant Parents.* Englewood Cliffs, New Jersey, Prentice-Hall, 1966.

Karmel, M.: *Thank You, Dr. Lamaze.* Philadelphia, J. B. Lippincott Company, 1959. (Paperback, Dolphin Books, Doubleday and Company, Inc., New York, 1965.) (Experiences of a mother with psychoprophylaxis.)

Pohl, M. L.: *Teaching Function of the Nursing Practitioner.* Iowa, William C. Brown Company Publishers, 1968.

Psychophysical Preparation for Childbearing: Guidelines for Teaching. 2nd Ed. New York, Maternity Center Association, 1965.

Shoemaker, L. P.: *Parent and Family-Life Education for Low-Income Families: A Guide for Leaders.* Children's Bureau Publication 434. Washington, D.C., U.S. Government Printing Office, U.S. Department of Health, Education and Welfare, 1965.

Vellay, P.: *Childbirth with Confidence,* pp. 46-66. New York, The Macmillan Company, 1965. (Sexual development and sex education.)

Wiedenbach, E.: *Family-Centered Maternity Nursing.* 2nd Ed., pp. 186-191. New York, G. P. Putnam's Sons, 1967. (Education for childbirth and parenthood.)

Ziegel, E., and Van Blarcom, C. C.: *Obstetric Nursing.* 5th Ed., pp. 132-137, 270-273. New York, The Macmillan Company, 1965.

JOURNAL ARTICLES

Abbott, F. E.: "Discussion Approach to Parent Group Education." *Childbirth Education,* 2:9, Winter 1969. (The meaning of discussion; class planning and content.)

Auerbach, A. B.: "Meeting the Needs of New Mothers." *Children,* 11:223, November-December 1964. (Includes feelings and fears of parents during pregnancy and puerperium; needs for education.)

Auerbach, A. B., and Rabinow, M.: "Parent Education Groups for Unmarried Mothers." *Nursing Outlook,* 14:38, March 1966. (Goals and content for classes for unwed mothers; nurses' feelings about working with unwed women.)

Beebe, J. E., et al.: "Bench Conferences in a Large Obstetric Clinic." *American Journal of Nursing,* 68:85, January 1968. (Method of disseminating knowledge in preparation for childbearing through informal, unstructured group interaction.)

Bruce, S. J.: "Do Prenatal Educational Programs Really Prepare for Parenthood?" *Hospital Topics,* 43:104, November 1965. (Types of programs; problems in planning; philosophy and goals of educational programs.)

Cochran, M. L., and Yeaworth, R. C.: "Ward Meetings for Teen-age Mothers." *American Journal of Nursing,* 67:1044, May 1967. (Overview and evaluation of group meetings conducted by nurses with young mothers on a hospital maternity unit.)

Conant, L. H.: "What Helps Mothers to Speak Out?" *American Journal of Nursing,* 69:2650, December 1969. (Study of factors influencing interaction patterns in child health conferences.)

Fitch, F. R.: "Sex Education for Mothers-to-Be." *The Bulletin of Maternal and Child Health,* 1:27, Winter 1965. (Suggestions for sex education of the new mother and the child, beginning in infancy. Types of questions children ask.)

Hogan, A.: "Launching Programs for Expectant Parents." *American Journal of Nursing,* 66:2227, October 1966. (Process of planning how, what, when, where and who to teach.)
Kariel, P. E.: "Social Class, Age, and Educational Group Differences in Childbirth Information." *Marriage and Family Living,* 25:353, August, 1963. (Comparison of knowledge regarding childbirth of primiparas – wives of university students of higher socioeconomic status and the "medically indigent.")
Lenahan, M. J.: "Looking for Teaching Aids?" *Nursing Outlook,* 16:48, October 1968. (Suggestions on where and how to obtain literature.)
Leppert, P., and Williams, B.: "Birth Films May Miscarry." *American Journal of Nursing,* 68:2181, October 1968. (Effects of birth films on expectant parents; suggestions for use of films; raises questions regarding use of films.)
McCaffery, M. S.: "An Approach to Parent Education." *Nursing Forum,* 6:1:77, 1967.
McCord, G.: "Public Health Assessess Childbirth Education." *Childbirth Education,* 3:2, Winter 1970. (Goals of childbirth education; raises questions about content and methodology of classes.)
Mohammed, M. F. B.: "Patients' Understanding of Written Health Information." *Nursing Research,* 13:100, Spring 1964.
Moore, B. M.: "Education for Family Living – What Is It?" *Nursing Clinics of North America,* 4:359, June 1969. (Components of family education, including sex education, family planning, family functions. Families with differing needs. Implications for nursing.)
Runnerstrom, L.: "Expectant Parent Education." *Nursing Science,* 3:57, February 1965. (Preparation beginning at an early age; groups developing educational programs; considerations in planning classes; overview of classes.)
Semmens, J. P.: "What the Schools Can and Should Teach in a Program of Family Life Education." *Obstetrics and Gynecology,* 28:723, November 1966. (Family life education beginning in infancy.)
Thaxton, A.: "Teaching Expectant Parents What They Want to Know." *American Journal of Nursing,* 62:112, May 1962. (Unstructured prenatal classes for parents; subjects covered; nurse's role.)
Treat, D. B.: "Understanding the Expectant Father." *Child and Family,* 3:16, Winter 1964. (Classes for expectant fathers; team teaching for couples' classes.)
Ulin, P. R.: "Changing Techniques in Psychoprophylactic Preparation for Childbirth." *American Journal of Nursing,* 68:2587, December 1968.
Yankauer, A., et al.: "What Mothers Say about Childbearing and Parents' Classes." *Nursing Outlook,* 8:563, October 1960. (Interviews with 283 mothers; their reactions to classes; implications for planning classes.)

OTHER PUBLICATIONS

Auerbach, A. B., and Arnstein, H. S.: *Pregnancy and You.* Child Study Association, 1962.
Children's Bureau: *Eat Well for You and Your Baby Who Is on the Way.* Washington, D.C., U.S. Government Printing Office, U.S. Department of Health, Education and Welfare, 1969.
Children's Bureau: *Prenatal Care.* Washington, D.C., U.S. Government Printing Office, U.S. Department of Health, Education and Welfare, 1962.
Children's Bureau: *When Your Baby Is on the Way.* Washington, D.C., U.S. Department of Health, Education and Welfare, 1961.
Dickinson-Belskie: *Birth Atlas.* 5th Ed. New York, Maternity Center Association, 1968.
Ross Laboratories: "Anticipatory Guidance." *Currents in Public Health.* Vol. 3, Number 4, April 1963.

NOTES

Guide 7

AMY WONDER'S FIRST STAGE OF LABOR

Amy and Harold Wonder arrive at the hospital at 2 A.M. Amy is expecting her first baby. Amy says her contractions began about six hours ago; they are now strong, regular and approximately five to seven minutes apart. She is sitting in a wheelchair holding her husband's hand when you first meet her. She is smiling and joking with another nurse.

1. Amy tells you she nearly came in a few days ago and was very disappointed "when it turned out to be only false labor." Differentiate between false labor and true labor.

2. Amy has been in labor for six hours when she enters the hospital. Her cervix is partially effaced and dilated 1 cm.

   a. What is effacement of the cervix?

b. What causes cervical effacement?

c. What is dilatation of the cervix?

d. What causes cervical dilatation?

e. How do the processes of dilatation and effacement differ in a primagravida and in a multigravida?

3. Amy is now in the first stage of labor.

   a. Briefly describe the three stages of labor.

b. State how long each stage generally lasts for a:

1) Primigravida

2) Multigravida

4. It is necessary to assess Amy's status immediately upon admission.

a. State the information you wish to obtain from Amy on admission.

b. State the observations you will make as you admit Amy to the labor room.

c. In what ways can the nurse be supportive to Amy during the admission procedure?

The following information is available on Amy's chart:

PRENATAL HISTORY AND ASSESSMENT SUMMARY

Name: Amy Wonder Age: 23 Marital Status: (M) S W D

Menstrual Onset: 12½ years, 28-day cycle, 4 days, moderate flow

Gravida: 1 Para: 0

Medical History: Normal childhood diseases

Surgical History: No surgeries

Physical Examination: Uterine pregnancy progressing normally

Pelvis adequate

BP 122/78

Usual weight: 120 pounds

Present weight: 138 pounds

Total weight gain: 18 pounds

Family history: Not significant

L. M. P.	January 10	Wasserman:	Neg.
E. D. C.	October 17	Urine:	sugar- neg.
			albumin- neg.
Fetal life felt:	June 1	Hemoglobin:	12.5%
Complications:	None	Blood Type:	O
		Rh:	positive

5. What information on this prenatal record is necessary in terms of providing nursing care to Amy? Why?

6. Amy's pelvic measurements are listed on the chart below.

   a. For each of these measurements state:

      1) Its abbreviation

      2) Whether it is an internal or external measurement

      3) How it is measured (estimated, pelvimeter, fingers, x-ray)

      4) The landmarks which describe the measurement

MEASUREMENTS	*ABBREVIATION*	*INTERNAL OR EXTERNAL*	*HOW MEASURED*	*LANDMARKS*
Intercristal 28 cm				
Interspinous 25 cm				
Intertrochanteric 31 cm				
External conjugate 19 cm				
Diagonal conjugate 12.5 cm				
True conjugate 11 cm				

MEASUREMENTS	*ABBREVIATION*	*INTERNAL OR EXTERNAL*	*HOW MEASURED*	*LANDMARKS*
Intertuberous diameter 8.5 cm				

b. State which of these measurements are considered most important in terms of the birth process.

7. a. Amy has a normal female pelvis. This is classified as a ____________ type of pelvis.

b. List the other three types of pelves.

c. State the significance of each of these pelvis types to the birth process.

8. Amy's prenatal summary indicates that her pelvis is adequate for vaginal delivery of her baby.

   a. Differentiate between the true pelvis and the false pelvis.

   b. Refer to the appropriate pictures and diagrams in a textbook and on the chart below, state:

      1) Obstetrical landmarks which indicate the true and the false pelvis

      2) Adaptations made by the baby in progressing through each of these landmarks

	OBSTETRICAL LANDMARKS	*ADAPTATION MADE BY BABY*
False pelvis		
True pelvis		
Inlet		
Mid-pelvis		

	OBSTETRICAL LANDMARKS	*ADAPTATION MADE BY BABY*
Outlet		

9. The adaptations Amy's baby makes as it descends through the birth canal are called the "mechanisms of labor."

   a. Differentiate between floating and engagement.

   b. What is the birth canal?

   c. Describe the four positional changes which constitute the mechanisms of labor.

d. Why is it necessary for these positional changes to occur?

10. State the significance, in terms of nursing care, of each of these notations on Amy's admission record:

Admission date and time: October 16, 2 A.M.

Membranes: intact

Contractions: 5–7 minutes, mild; approximately 6 hours' duration

No show

FHT: LLQ regular 130

Station: -1

Dilatation: 1 cm

Last meal: Supper: October 15 at 6 P.M., soup and sandwich

Comments: Attended parents' classes with husband
Familiar with psychoprophylaxis
Husband to be with her during labor and delivery

11. Amy may have clear fluids but no food during the early part of her labor.

    a. What is the physiological reason for restricting food during Amy's labor?

b. Why are clear fluids permitted only during the early first stage of Amy's labor?

12. When Amy is settled in the labor room, you prepare her for the enema and perineal shave which have been ordered.

    a. Why might an enema be ordered prior to delivery?

    b. State the principles you will follow when administering the enema.

    c. Under what circumstances would an enema be contraindicated?

13. Amy is to have her perineum shaved.

    a. What is the purpose of this procedure?

b. State the principles you will follow while shaving Amy's perineum.

c. In some institutions, an obstetrician may order either a perineal shave or a vulvar shave, or no shave may be carried out. What are the pros and cons of these procedures?

14. Amy's obstetrician may do either a rectal or vaginal examination to determine the progress of her labor. Nurses perform these examinations in some institutions.

a. State, specifically, what can be determined by each of these examinations.

b. What are the current thoughts concerning the performance of vaginal examinations by nurses?

c. What are the current thoughts concerning the performance of rectal examinations by nurses?

15. Amy's husband is timing her contractions along with you.

a. What are Amy's contractions accomplishing?

b. Describe the characteristics of mild, moderate and strong contractions.

c. State, specifically, the change to be expected in the duration and intensity of Amy's contractions during this first stage of labor.

d. You have asked Harold to time Amy's contractions. Why?

16. Amy is in the first stage of labor. For each of the three phases of this stage, state the:

a. Behavioral characteristics you can anticipate with Amy

b. Physical and emotional support Harold can give Amy

c. Physical and emotional support the nurse can give Amy (be sure to include instructions related to breathing)

d. Support the nurse can give Harold during this time

e. The nurse's responsibilities, other than support during each phase of the first stage of labor

(Use chart on next page)

	FIRST PHASE (Early First Stage)	*SECOND PHASE (Late First Stage)*	*THIRD PHASE (Transitional)*
Amy's behavioral characteristics			
Support Harold can give to Amy			
Support Nurse can give to Amy			

	FIRST PHASE (Early First Stage)	*SECOND PHASE (Late First Stage)*	*THIRD PHASE (Transitional)*
Support Nurse can give to Harold			
Nurse's additional responsibilities			

17. What instructions will you give Amy when she wants to "push" during and in between each contraction?

18. You listen to the fetal heart tones with a fetascope and note the rate is 138 beats per minute and regular.

   a. 1) How do you determine the location of the fetal heart tones?

2) What information from Amy's chart will be helpful to you?

b. What is the normal range for the fetal heart rate?

c. What is the significance of a fetal heart rate which is above or below this range? What implications does this have for nursing?

d. You may hear uterine souffle or funic souffle.

1) What is uterine souffle?

2) What is funic souffle?

e. Would you suggest that Amy and Harold listen to their baby's fetal heart tones? Why?

f. What other methods are used for monitoring the fetal heart rate?

19. a. At 5 A.M., Amy's membranes rupture. State your nursing responsibilities at this time and the rationale for each action you will take.

b. State your nursing responsibilities if prolapse of the umbilical cord should occur. State the rationale for each action.

20. Amy received meperidine hydrochloride (Demerol) 50 mg IM during the latter half of the first stage of labor. There are other medications a woman in labor might receive. For each of the medications listed below, state:

a. The usual dosage

b. The expected physiological action

c. Untoward effects on the mother or baby

d. Nursing observations or measures indicated

DRUG	*DOSAGE*	*PHYSIOLOGICAL ACTION*	*UNTOWARD EFFECTS*		*NURSING IMPLICATIONS*
			MOTHER	*BABY*	
Hydroxyzine pamoate (Vistaril)					

DRUG	*DOSAGE*	*PHYSIOLOGICAL ACTION*	*UNTOWARD EFFECTS MOTHER*	*BABY*	*NURSING IMPLICATIONS*
Meperidine hydrochloride (Demerol)					
Morphine sulfate					
Oxytocin (Pitocin)					
Promethazine (Phenergan)					

DRUG	DOSAGE	PHYSIOLOGICAL ACTION	UNTOWARD EFFECTS MOTHER	BABY	NURSING IMPLICATIONS
Scopolamine hydrobromide					
Sodium seconal					

21. What drugs may be used in combination with each other during labor?

REFERENCES

BOOKS

Barnes, A. C.: "Prevention of Congenital Anomalies from the Point of View of the Obstetrician." *Congenital Malformations,* International Medical Congress, Limited, 1964. (Genetic counseling; prenatal care; maternal disease; pregnancy-related diseases; labor and delivery.)

Bergersen, B. S., and Krug, E. E.: *Pharmacology In Nursing.* 11th Ed. St. Louis, The C. V. Mosby Company, 1969.

Bing, E. D. (Ed.): *The Adventure of Birth.* New York, Simon and Schuster, 1970. (Accounts by mothers and fathers of their experience with the Lamaze method of childbirth.)

Bookmiller, M. M., et al.: *Textbook of Obstetrics and Obstetric Nursing.* 5th Ed. Philadelphia, W. B. Saunders Company, 1967.

Bryant, R. D., and Overland, A. E.: *Obstetric Management and Nursing.* 7th Ed. Philadelphia, F. A. Davis Company, 1964. (Baptism.)

Buxton, C. L.: *A Study of Psychophysical Methods of Relief of Childbirth Pain.* Philadelphia, W. B. Saunders Company, 1962. (Natural childbirth; hypnosis; education.)

Chabon, I.: *Awake and Aware: Participating in Childbirth Through Prophylaxis.* New York, Delacorte Press, 1966. (Paperback, New York, Dell Publishing Company, Inc. 1969.)

Dally, A., and Sweering, R.: *The Birth of a Child.* New York, Crown Publishers, Inc., 1969. (Written and pictorial description of the normal birth process.)

Eastman, N. J., and Hellman, L. M.: *Williams Obstetrics.* 12th Ed., pp. 281-336, 373-441. New York, Appleton-Century-Crofts, Inc., 1961.
Fuerst, E. V., and Wolff, L.: *Fundamentals of Nursing.* 4th Ed. Philadelphia, J. B. Lippincott Company, 1969.
Guyton, A. C.: *Textbook of Medical Physiology.* 3rd Ed., pp. 1153-1159. Philadelphia, W. B. Saunders Company, 1966.
Huntingford, P. J., et al. (Eds.): *Perinatal Medicine.* New York, Academic Press, 1969. (Amniotic fluid analysis; prevention, diagnosis and treatment of Rh incompatibility; electronic fetal heart monitoring; fetal blood sampling; clinical relationships between mother and fetus during labor; resuscitation of newborn; high risk baby; treatment of respiratory disturbances in newborn.)
Jacob, S. W., and Francone, C. A.: *Structure and Function in Man.* 2nd Ed. Philadelphia, W. B. Saunders Company, 1970.
Karmel, M.: *Thank You, Dr. Lamaze.* Philadelphia, J. B. Lippincott Company, 1959. (Paperback, Dolphin Books, Doubleday and Company, Inc., New York, 1965.) (Experiences of a mother with psychoprophylaxis.)
Kozier, B. B., and DuGas, B. W.: *Fundamentals of Patient Care.* Philadelphia, W. B. Saunders Company, 1967.
Manual of Standards in Obstetric-Gynecologic Practice. 2nd Ed. Chicago, The American College of Obstetricians and Gynecologists, 1965.
Maternity Center Association: *A Baby Is Born.* Revised Ed. New York, Maternity Center Association, 1964.
Rodman, M. J., and Smith, D. W.: *Pharmacology and Drug Therapy in Nursing.* Philadelphia, J. B. Lippincott Company, 1968.
Wiedenbach, E.: *Family-Centered Maternity Care.* 2nd Ed. New York, G. P. Putnam's Sons, 1967.
Ziegel, E., and Van Blarcom, C. C.: *Obstetric Nursing.* 5th Ed., pp. 201-255. New York, The Macmillan Company, 1965.

JOURNAL ARTICLES

Allen, S.: "Nurse Attendance During Labor." *American Journal of Nursing,* 64:70, June 1964. (Effects of nurse attendance during labor; induction of labor; amniocentesis; suggestions for nursing intervention.)
Attoway, J. P.: "Vaginal vs. Rectal Examinations in Evaluation of Labor Status." *Hospital Topics,* 45:101, March 1967.
Danforth, D. N., and Baldwin, C. A.: "Pain Relief in the Parturient." *Medical Clinics of North America,* 52:137, January 1968. (Indications for analgesia; techniques of analgesia and anesthesia; effects on mother and fetus; hypnosis and natural childbirth.)
Friedman, E. A.: "Relation of Maternal Age to the Course of Labor." *American Journal of Obstetrics and Gynecology,* 91:915, April 1, 1965.
Hannah, W. J.: "The Use of Oxytocin in Obstetrics." *Applied Therapeutics,* 11:216, April 1969. (Physiological action; indications for use – antepartum, intrapartum, postpartum – methods of administration; abuses and hazards.)
Hilmar, N.: "Standards and Criteria as Health Protection Tools." *American Journal of Public Health,* 59:1613, September 1969. (Governmental responsibility to establish and promote health protection standards.)
Larsen, V. L.: "Stresses of the Childbearing Year." *American Journal of Public Health,* 56:32, January 1966. (Stresses during pregnancy, labor and delivery; postpartum and first three months at home.)
Long, A. E.: "The Unshaved Perineum at Parturition." *American Journal of Obstetrics and Gynecology,* 99:333, October 1, 1967.
Matousek, I.: "Fetal Nursing During Labor." *Nursing Clinics of North America,* 3:307, June 1968. (Proposed routine for fetal nursing; importance of mother and fetal assessment and care.)
McCain, F. R.: "Nursing by Assessment – Not Intuition." *American Journal of Nursing,* 65:82, April 1965.
Tryon, P. A.: "Assessing the Progress of Labor Through Observation of Patients' Behavior." *Nursing Clinics of North America,* 3:315, June 1968.
Ueland, K., and Hansen, J. M.: "Maternal Cardiovascular Dynamics, II. Posture and Uterine Contractions." *American Journal of Obstetrics and Gynecology,* 103:1, January 1, 1969.

OTHER PUBLICATIONS

Bonica, J. J.: *An Atlas on Mechanisms and Pathways of Pain in Labor.* North Chicago, Abbott Laboratories, Spring 1960.
Dickinson-Belskie: *Birth Atlas.* 5th Ed. New York, Maternity Center Association, 1968.
Rose, P. A.: "Identification and Application of Psychiatric Principles in the Nursing Care of Maternity Patients." *Phases in Human Development: Relevance in Nursing,* ANA 1962 Clinical Sessions, 10 Columbus Circle, New York. (Detailed analysis of a nurse's interaction with a 19-year-old primipara during labor, delivery and postpartum; some interaction with husband.)

NOTES

Guide 8

AMY WONDER'S SECOND AND THIRD STAGES OF LABOR

PART I. AMY WONDER'S SECOND STAGE OF LABOR

Amy Wonder, a primigravida with an uncomplicated pregnancy, has been in the first stage of labor for nine hours. Her husband, Harold, has been with her throughout the labor. When checking Amy's perineum, you had noted bulging. Now you note the baby's head begins to crown.

1. What does crowning of the baby's head indicate?

2. Amy is moved to the delivery room, accompanied by Harold.

    a. What will be Harold's role during the delivery?

    b. What is the nurse's role in relation to Harold?

c. If Harold was not permitted in the delivery room:

1) What might be his possible thoughts and feelings while waiting for the delivery?

2) What could the nurse do to support him during the waiting period?

3. Amy will be placed in a lithotomy position for delivery. What factors must the nurse consider in positioning and preparing Amy for the delivery now that she is in the delivery room?

4. Amy's hands will not be restrained during the delivery.

a. Under what circumstances is it necessary to restrain a woman's hands?

b. What instructions will you give Amy in relation to her hands?

5. Because it is the nurse's responsibility, you have checked to see that the delivery room is set up for Amy's delivery. What equipment would you be certain is readily available when you bring Amy into the room?

6. Amy said she wanted to be awake for the delivery of her baby, but she does want a local anesthetic. She was confused about various types of nerve block anesthesia before they were explained to her. For each of the types of administration listed below, state the:

   a. Area which is anesthetized

   b. Method of administration

   c. Nursing implications prior to, during, and following administration

TYPE	*AREA*	*METHOD*	*NURSING IMPLICATIONS*		
			BEFORE	*DURING*	*AFTER*
Spinal					
Saddle block					
Caudal					

TYPE	*AREA*	*METHOD*	*NURSING IMPLICATIONS* *BEFORE*	*DURING*	*AFTER*
Pudendal block					
Local infiltration					

d. What medications are generally administered for nerve block anesthesia?

7. Amy will be awake during the delivery and wants to observe the birth of her baby.

   a. State the nurse's role in supporting Amy during the delivery.

   b. State the nursing observations made during the delivery in relation to:

      1) Amy

      2) The baby

      3) Harold

8. Amy did not want a general anesthetic for her delivery. However, because general anesthetics are used during delivery, you must be knowledgeable about the various types. For each of the following anesthetics, state the:

   a. Route of administration

b. Effects on mother and fetus

c. Contraindications

d. Nurse's care of the mother and fetus during and following administration

ANESTHETIC	ROUTE	EFFECTS		CONTRA-INDICATIONS	NURSING CARE
		MOTHER	FETUS		
Chloroform					
Cyclopropane					
Ether					
Nitrous oxide and oxygen					

ANESTHETIC	ROUTE	EFFECTS MOTHER	EFFECTS FETUS	CONTRA-INDICATIONS	NURSING CARE
Thiopental sodium (Sodium Pentothal)					
Trichlro-ethylene (Trilene)					

9. Two drugs which reverse the effects of analgesics and anesthetics are nalorphine hydrochloride (Nalline) and caffeine sodium benzoate. For each of these medications, state:

   a. Its action

   b. The route of administration

   c. Who will receive the drug (mother or baby)

   d. When the drug is to be administered
   (Chart on page 141)

	NALORPHINE HYDROCHLORIDE (NALLINE)	*CAFFEINE SODIUM BENZOATE*
Action of drug		
Route of administration		
Received by mother or baby		
When administered		

10. What is the nurse's responsibility to the physician during the delivery?

11. Amy may be catheterized before the delivery. Why would this be necessary?

12. The lie, presentation and position of Amy's baby is "left occiput anterior."

    a. What is the abbreviation for this presentation?

    b. Below are other designations of presentations. For each presentation, state the:

        1) Presenting part and position

        2) Implications of each of these presentations in terms of labor and delivery

            (a) R.O.A.

            (b) L.M.P.

            (c) L.O.P.

            (d) R.S.A.

            (e) L.Sc.A.

13. Amy's obstetrician performs a mediolateral episiotomy.

    a. What other type of episiotomy might have been performed?

    b. Differentiate between these two types of episiotomy.

THE BABY IS DELIVERED AND IT IS A BOY!

14. What reactions might Amy and Harold have?

15. What reactions might the nurse have?

16. Amy sustained no lacerations during the delivery.

    a. Why do lacerations occur during the delivery?

b. Differentiate between a first, second and third degree laceration.

17. The use of forceps or a vacuum extractor was not necessary during Amy's delivery.

   a. What are the indications for the use of forceps during delivery of a baby?

   b. Differentiate between high and low forceps application during delivery.

   c. State the knowledges you would need in order to discuss with a mother the forceps marks on her infant's head.

   d. What is vacuum extraction?

   e. Describe the appearance of an infant's head following vacuum extraction.

18. Amy's labor and delivery were considered "normal." She was attended by her husband, obstetrician and nurse. Assuming her labor had progressed more rapidly than anticipated and the obstetrician had not been available for the delivery, state the activities you would have carried out in delivering the infant and state the rationale for each.

PART II. AMY WONDER'S THIRD STAGE OF LABOR

19. What are the nurse's responsibilities to Amy immediately following the delivery of the baby?

20. After delivery of the placenta, the physician says, "The placenta is delivered as Schultz and is intact."

    a. What does this statement mean?

    b. What are the significant differences between the Duncan and the Schultz methods of delivery of the placenta?

    c. State the nurse's responsibility to Amy immediately following delivery of the placenta.

21. The baby is put to Amy's breast while she is still on the delivery table and nurses for about two minutes. State the the advantages of this to:

    a. Amy

    b. The baby

22. Amy received methergine 0.2 mg IM in the delivery room.

    a. Name at least three other oxytocics which may be given instead of methergine.

    b. State the action of these medications.

    c. State the advantages and disadvantages of these medications.

23. Amy and Harold hold their new son, David, while they are in the delivery room. What are the advantages of this initial contact?

24. Following the delivery, Amy's legs are simultaneously lowered from the stirrups. Why are both legs lowered at the same time?

25. What are your nursing responsibilities to Amy before she leaves the delivery room?

REFERENCES

BOOKS

Barnes, A. C.: "Prevention of Congenital Anomalies from the Point of View of the Obstetrician." *Congenital Malformations,* International Medical Congress, Limited, 1964. (Genetic counseling; prenatal care; maternal disease; pregnancy-related diseases; labor and delivery.)

Bergersen, B. S., and Krug, E. E.: *Pharmacology In Nursing.* 11th Ed. St. Louis, The C. V. Mosby Company, 1969.

Bing, E. D. (Ed.): *The Adventure of Birth.* New York, Simon and Schuster, 1970. (Accounts by mothers and fathers of their experience with the Lamaze method of childbirth.)

Bookmiller, M. M., et al.: *Textbook of Obstetric Nursing.* 5th Ed. Philadelphia, W. B. Saunders Company, 1967.

Bryant, R. D., and Overland, A. E.: *Obstetric Management and Nursing.* 7th Ed. Philadelphia, F. A. Davis Company, 1964. (Baptism.)

Buxton, C. L.: *A Study of Psychophysical Methods of Relief of Childbirth Pain.* Philadelphia, W. B. Saunders Company, 1962. (Natural childbirth; hypnosis; education.)

Chabon, I.: *Awake and Aware: Participating in Childbirth Through Prophylaxis.* New York, Delacorte Press, 1966. (Paperback, New York, Dell Publishing Company, Inc., 1969.)

Dally, A., and Sweering, R.: *The Birth of a Child.* New York, Crown Publishers, Inc., 1969. (Written and pictorial description of the normal birth process.)

Eastman, N. J., and Hellman, L. M.: *Williams Obstetrics.* 12th Ed., pp. 441-490. New York, Appleton-Century-Crofts, Inc., 1961.

Fuerst, E. V., and Wolff, L.: *Fundamentals of Nursing.* 4th Ed. Philadelphia, J. B. Lippincott Company, 1969.

Grimm, E. R.: "Psychological and Social Factors in Pregnancy, Delivery, and Outcome." In Richardson, S. A., and Guttmacher, A. F. (Eds.): *Childbearing – Its Social and Psychological Aspects,* pp. 1-52. Baltimore, The Williams and Wilkins Company, 1967.

Guyton, A. C.: *Textbook of Medical Physiology.* 3rd Ed., pp. 1153-1159. Philadelphia, W. B. Saunders Company, 1966.

Jacob, S. W., and Francone, C. A.: *Structure and Function in Man.* 2nd Ed. Philadelphia, W. B. Saunders Company, 1970.
Kozier, B. B. and DuGas, B. W.: *Fundamentals of Patient Care.* Philadelphia, W. B. Saunders Company, 1967.
Maternity Center Association: *A Baby Is Born.* Revised Ed. New York, Maternity Center Association, 1964.
Nesbitt, R. E. L.: "Primary Prevention from the Viewpoint of the Obstetrician." In Lytle, N. A.: *Maternal Health Nursing,* pp. 31-49. Iowa, William C. Brown Company, Inc., 1967. (Prenatal care; prematurity; third trimester bleeding; fetal distress; toxemia, labor.)
Rodman, M. J., and Smith, D. W.: *Pharmacology and Drug Therapy in Nursing.* Philadelphia, J. B. Lippincott Company, 1968.
Shnider, S. M. (Ed.): *Obstetrical Anesthesia: Current Concepts and Practices.* Baltimore, The Williams and Wilkins Company, 1970.
Wiedenbach, E.: *Family-Centered Maternity Care.* 2nd Ed. New York, G. P. Putnam's Sons, 1967.
Ziegel, E., and Van Blarcom, C. C.: *Obstetric Nursing.* 5th Ed., pp. 255-365, 269-284. New York, The Macmillan Company, 1965.

JOURNAL ARTICLES

Adriani, J.: "Obstetric Analgesia and Anesthesia." *American Family Physician/GP,* 1:66, March 1970. (Types of anesthesia – general and regional; types and techniques of analgesia.)
Alexander, L.: "Rectals and Vaginals: The OB Nurse's Job?" *Registered Nurse,* 29:39, February 1966.
Allen, S.: "Nurse Attendance During Labor." *American Journal of Nursing,* 64:70, June 1964. (Effects of nurse attendance during labor; induction of labor; amniocentesis; suggestions for nursing intervention.)
Danforth, D. N., and Baldwin, C. A.: "Pain Relief in the Parturient." *Medical Clinics of North America,* 52:137, January 1968. (Indications for analgesia; techniques of analgesia and anesthesia; effects on mother and fetus; hypnosis and "natural childbirth.")
Goldstein, J.: "Exploring Attitudes that Affect Nursing Care." *Nursing Outlook,* 16:50, June 1968. (Attitudes of practical nursing students toward death and birth.)
Hannah, W. J.: "The Use of Oxytocin in Obstetrics." *Applied Therapeutics,* 11:216, April 1969. (Physiological action; indications for use – antepartum, intrapartum, postpartum; methods of administration; abuses and hazards)
Hoff, F. E.: "Natural Childbirth, How Any Nurse Can Help." *American Journal of Nursing,* 69:1451, July 1969. (Overview of physical and emotional supportive measures of the nurse.)
Larsen, V. L.: "Stresses of the Childbearing Year." *American Journal of Public Health,* 56:32, January 1966. (Stresses during pregnancy, labor and delivery, postpartum and first three months at home.)
Melber, R.: "The Nurse's Role in Obstetrical Emergencies in the Hospital Setting." *Nursing Clinics of North America,* 2:261, June 1967. (Preparation for and when emergency occurs.)
Tryon, P. A.: "Assessing the Progress of Labor Through Observation of Patients' Behavior." *Nursing Clinics of North America,* 3:315, June 1968.
Ueland, K., and Hansen, J. M.: "Maternal Cardiovascular Dynamics, III. Labor and Delivery Under Local and Caudal Analgesia." *American Journal of Obstetrics and Gynecology,* 103:8, January 1, 1969.

OTHER PUBLICATIONS

Dickinson-Belskie: *Birth Atlas.* 5th Ed. New York, Maternity Center Association.
Rose, P. A.: "Identification and Application of Psychiatric Principles in the Nursing Care of Maternity Patients." *Phases in Human Development: Relevance in Nursing,* ANA 1962 Clinical Sessions, 10 Columbus Circle, New York, pp. 14-36. (Detailed analysis of a nurse's interaction with a 19-year-old primipara during labor, delivery and postpartum; some interaction with husband.)
Ross Laboratories: *Obstetrical Presentation and Position.* Columbus, Ohio, 1958.
Ross Laboratories: *Phenomena of Normal Labor.* Columbus, Ohio, 1964.

NOTES

Guide 9

DAVID WONDER ADAPTS TO HIS NEW SURROUNDINGS

PART I. CARE OF DAVID IMMEDIATELY FOLLOWING DELIVERY

1. What measures are taken to clear David's air passages as soon as he is born?

2. Why is David placed with his head down after birth?

3. David cries spontaneously. If he did not cry spontaneously, how would he be stimulated to cry?

4. David needs suctioning to remove some mucus.

   a. State the principles to follow while suctioning him.

   b. State three types of suction apparatus which are available for suctioning newborn infants. How do they differ?

5. David does not need to be resuscitated. However, you must know how to resuscitate an infant when necessary. State:

   a. The indications for resuscitation of a newborn infant following delivery

   b. The principles to follow when resuscitating an infant

c. How resuscitation is performed

d. Equipment and medications which should be available in the delivery room for resuscitation

e. A brief description of asphyxia neonatorum

6. If David's heart had failed to beat, closed chest cardiac massage would have been initiated.

a. State the principles of external cardiac massage of a newborn infant.

b. How is external cardiac massage of a newborn infant performed?

7. Under what circumstances would you baptize a newborn infant?

8. You observe David's cord and note that it has three vessels.

   a. What are these vessels?

   b. What would be the significance of a cord with two vessels?

9. David's Apgar score is recorded 60 seconds after birth. His score is 9 and is distributed as follows:

Heart rate	2
Respiratory effort	2
Muscle tone	2
Reflex irritability	2
Color	1

   a. On the chart on page 157, state:

      1) The meaning of a score of 0, 1 and 2 related to each of the signs

      2) How each sign is determined

SIGN	*APGAR SCORE* 0	1	2	*HOW DETERMINED*
Heart rate				
Respiratory effort				
Muscle tone				
Reflex irritability				
Color				

b. State the significance of:

1) David's Apgar score of 9

2) An Apgar score of 5

3) An Apgar score of 2

10. How does the temperature in the delivery room differ from David's environmental temperature in utero? What implications does this have for David's immediate care following birth?

11. David Wonder is to receive 1 per cent silver nitrate eye drops followed by irrigation with normal saline to prevent ophthalmia neonatorum.

    a. What is ophthalmia neonatorum?

    b. What other medications may be administered other than silver nitrate?

    c. How will you open David's eyes?

    d. What principles must be followed when instilling the eye medication?

    e. What is chemical conjunctivitis?

12. David is to receive an intramuscular injection of a vitamin K preparation.

    a. Why is vitamin K frequently given to newborn infants?

b. State the principles you will follow when administering an intramuscular injection to a newborn infant.

c. What site will you select for the injection? Why?

13. David is to be identified with two identification bands, one on his wrist and one on his ankle. An identical band is placed on Amy's wrist.

a. Why is it necessary to identify David Wonder immediately?

b. What other methods are used to identify newborn infants?

c. Why does Amy have an identification band identical to David's bands?

14. David is transferred to the transition nursery, where he will remain for 12 hours before being placed in Amy's room.

a. What are your responsibilities while transferring David from the delivery room to the nursery?

b. State the information you will give the nurse accepting David in the nursery.

PART II. DAVID'S ADAPTATION AND NURSING CARE

15. Approximately how long will it take David's systems to adapt to extrauterine life?

16. What factors will determine the success of David's neonatal adjustment?

17. What is the time span referred to as the neonatal period?

18. David takes his first breath almost immediately after his head is delivered.

    a. What factors are thought to play a role in the initiation of the first breath?

    b. How soon after birth do vigorous infants usually breathe?

c. State the physiological changes which occur when David takes his first breath.

d. Describe the expected rate and character of David's respirations during his first 24 hours of life.

e. What are your nursing responsibilities related to David's respiratory adaptation?

19. Simultaneously with David's first respiratory activity, changes are taking place within his circulatory system.

a. Review the circulation of the fetus (see Study Guide 5: Baby Wonder's Development, question 23, page 85).

b. State the anatomical changes which occur in David's circulatory system following his birth.

c. What determines David's total blood volume immediately following delivery?

d. What observations would indicate that David's peripheral circulation is sluggish after birth?

e. Why is David's peripheral circulation sluggish after birth?

f. Describe the expected characteristics of David's heart rate and rhythm.

g. How will you ascertain David's heart rate? Why?

h. What would you expect David's blood pressure to be?

i. Why do an infant's pulse and blood pressure differ from those of an adult?

j. What constitutes hematopoietic tissue in the:

1) fetus

2) infant

k. State the changes which will occur in the following blood constituents from the time of David's birth until he is approximately three months old.

1) Red blood cells

2) Hemoglobin

3) Bilirubin

4) White blood cells

l. Differentiate between fetal hemoglobin and adult hemoglobin.

m. When does the fetus begin to store iron?

n. When do infants lose their store of iron?

o. Newborn infants have a blood coagulation deficiency.

1) Why do newborn infants have a blood coagulation deficiency?

2) How long does it last?

3) How is it treated?

p. What are your nursing responsibilities related to David's circulatory system adjustments?

20. David's metabolic rate differs from that of his father.

a. How does David's metabolic rate differ from that of his father? Why?

b. State the implications this has in terms of:

1) Caloric requirements

2) Fluid requirements

21. You will be taking David's temperature when he arrives in the nursery.

a. Why will you take David's initial temperature rectally?

b. State the usual temperature range of newborn infants.

c. State the anatomical and physiological characteristics of a newborn infant which influence David's ability to regulate his temperature.

d. State the nursing responsibilities necessitated by David's immature temperature regulation.

22. David is more susceptible to infections than he will be in another year.

    a. Why are infants more susceptible to infections than older children and their parents?

    b. What factors influence the type of immunity an infant receives from his mother?

    c. What immunity does David receive from his mother?

    d. State the nursing principles and measures needed to protect David from infection while he is still in the hospital.

23. a. State the changes which will occur in David's gastrointestinal system during the neonatal period.

b. What implications do these gastrointestinal changes have for nursing care?

24. a. How soon after birth can David be expected to have a stool?

b. What would be the possible meaning of David's failure to have a stool within this time?

c. Describe David's first stool.

d. Describe the transitional stool. When does it occur?

e. Describe David's stools when he is one week old. He is being breast fed.

f. Describe the stools of a week-old bottle-fed infant.

25. a. What changes take place in David's kidney function following birth?

b. When can David be expected to void following birth?

c. What is the possible meaning of his failure to void within this period?

d. What nursing observations are necessitated by David's kidney functioning?

26. You weigh David and find that his birth weight is 7 pounds 2 ounces.

a. State the average birth weight in the United States for:

1) White infants

2) Nonwhite infants

3) Male infants

4) Female infants

b. What factors influence an infant's birth weight?

c. State the changes which can be expected in David's weight over the next two weeks.

27. David measures 19½ inches in length at birth. What is the average length of newborn infants?

REFERENCES

BOOKS

Abramson, H. (Ed.): *Resuscitation of the Newborn Infant.* 2nd Ed. St. Louis, The C. V. Mosby Company, 1966.

American Academy of Pediatrics: *Standards and Recommendations for Hospital Care of Newborn Infants.* Evanston, Illinois, 1964.

Bergersen, B. S., and Krug, E. E.: *Pharmacology in Nursing.* 11th Ed. St. Louis, The C. V. Mosby Company, 1969.

Blake, F. C., et al.: *Nursing Care of Children.* 8th Ed. Philadelphia, J. B. Lippincott Company, 1970.

Bryant, R. D., and Overland, A. E.: *Obstetric Management and Nursing.* 7th Ed. Philadelphia, F. A. Davis Company, 1964. (Baptism.)

Eastman, N. J., and Hellman, L. M.: *Williams Obstetrics.* 12th Ed., pp. 511-523. New York, Appleton-Century-Crofts, Inc., 1961.

Guyton, A. C.: *Textbook of Medical Physiology.* 3rd Ed. Philadelphia, W. B. Saunders Company, 1966.

Huntingford, P. J., et al. (Eds.): *Perinatal Medicine.* New York, Academic Press, 1969. (Amniotic fluid analysis; prevention, diagnosis and treatment of Rh incapability; electronic fetal heart monitoring; fetal blood sampling; clinical relationships between mother and fetus during labor; resuscitation of newborn; high risk baby; treatment of respiratory disturbances in newborn.)

Leifer, G.: *Principles and Techniques in Pediatric Nursing.* Philadelphia, W. B. Saunders Company, 1965.

Marlow, D. R.: *Textbook of Pediatric Nursing.* 3rd Ed. Philadelphia, W. B. Saunders Company, 1969.

McKilligan, H.: *The First Day of Life: Principles of Neonatal Nursing.* New York, Springer Publishing Company, Inc., 1970.

Rodman, M. J., and Smith, D. W.: *Pharmacology and Drug Therapy in Nursing.* Philadelphia, J. B. Lippincott Company, 1968.

Ziegel, E., and Van Blarcom, C. C.: *Obstetric Nursing.* 5th Ed., pp. 507-595. New York, The Macmillan Company, 1965.

JOURNAL ARTICLES

Apgar, V.: "Resuscitation of the Newborn: When and How to Do it." *Hospital Topics,* 44:105, November 1966. (Describes Apgar score; methods of resuscitation.)

Arnold, H. W., et al.: "The Newborn – Transition to Extra-uterine Life." *American Journal of Nursing,* 65:77, October 1965. (Excellent for bibliographies.)

Battaglia, F. C.: "Recent Advances in Medicine for Newborn Infants." *Journal of Pediatrics,* 71:748, November 1967. (Association of obstetric complications with neonatal problems; treatment of idiopathic respiratory distress syndrome; intrauterine growth retardation; neonatal metabolic complications.)

Berrien, C. D.: "Evaluating the Newborn." *Nursing Outlook,* 9:93, February 1961. (Performance and interpretation of Apgar score in the delivery room.)

Buchanan-Davidson, D. J.: "What We Can Learn from Meconium." *American Journal of Nursing,* 63:112, July 1963. (Description of normal and abnormal meconium.)

Desmond, M. M., et al.: "The Clinical Behavior of the Newly Born." *Journal of Pediatrics,* 62:307, March 1963. (General activity; autonomic activity; pulse and respiratory rates of newborn infants from birth to six hours.)

Drage, J. S., et al.: "The Apgar Score as an Index of Neonatal Mortality." *Obstetrics and Gynecology,* 24:222, August 1964.

Du, J. N. H., and Oliver, T. K., Jr.: "The Baby in the Delivery Room." *Journal of the American Medical Association,* 207:1502, February 24, 1969. (Use of radiant heat to control infant's temperature in delivery room.)

"Fetal Reaction to and Survival after Labor and Birth." *Child and Family,* 4:4, Fall 1965. (Intrauterine environment; effect of labor on infant; abnormal pregnancy and labor; normal newborn, complications of newborn period.)

James, L. S., et al.: "Respiratory Physiology of the Fetus and Newborn Infant." *New England Journal of Medicine,* 271:1403, December 31, 1964.

McKay, R. J., and Lucey, J. F.: "Neonatology." *The New England Journal of Medicine,* 270:1231, June 4, 1964. (Drugs; immunity; respiratory distress syndrome; infants of diabetic mothers; hypoglycemia.)

McKay, R. J., and Lucey, J. F.: "Neonatology." *The New England Journal of Medicine,* 270:1292, June 11, 1964. (Jaundice; twins; prematurity; aids to diagnosing neonatal disease.)

Oppé T. E.: "The Baby's Blood." *Nursing Mirror,* 129:17, August 15, 1969. (Normal and abnormal characteristics of red cells, white cells and platelets of fetus and newborn infant.)

Polgar, G.: "The First Breath: A Turbulent Period of Physiologic Adjustment." *Clinical Pediatrics,* 2:562, October 1963. (Anatomical development; respiratory center stimuli; process of delivery; entry of air into lungs; circulatory adjustments.)

Prystowsky, H.: "Intrauterine Growth and Development of the Baby." *Clinical Obstetrics and Gynecology,* 6:544, September 1963. (Fetal respiration; circulation, metabolic processes; neonatal blood counts; some abnormal neonatal conditions.)

Ravitch, M. M., and Rowe, M. I.: "Surgical Emergencies in the Neonate." *American Journal of Obstetrics and Gynecology,* 103:1034, April 1, 1969.

Rudolph, A. M.: "The Changes in Circulation after Birth." *Circulation,* 41:343, February 1970. (Good diagrams.)

Silverman, W. A.: "Diagnosis and Treatment: Use and Misuse of Temperature and Humidity in Care of Newborn Infant." *Pediatrics,* 33:276, February 1964.

Sinclair, J. C.: "Heat Production and Thermo-regulation in the Small-for-Date Infant." *Pediatric Clinics of North America,* 17:147, February 1970. (Heat production and dissipation; physiological responses to heat and cold; clinical consequences of cold stress of small-for-date and full-term infants.)

Smith, C. A.: "The First Breath." *Scientific American,* 209:27, October 1963.

Tancer, M. L., et al.: "Group A, Type 33, B-hemolytic, Streptococcal Outbreak on a Maternity and Newborn Service." *American Journal of Obstetrics and Gynecology,* 103:1028, April 1, 1969. (Recognition and control of an infection; recommendations for prevention, early recognition and control.)

Wells, J.: "Effect on the Newborn of Induced Versus Spontaneous Labor." *Obstetrics and Gynecology,* 26:580, October 1965.

Whitner, W., and Thompson, M. C.: "The Influence of Bathing on the Newborn Infant's Body Temperature." *Nursing Research,* 19:30, January-February 1970.

Wright, E. J., and Lewis, R. L.: "Treating the Newborn as a Recovering Patient." *Hospital Topics,* 45:93, October 1967. (Nurses' role in caring for newborn infant in nursery.)

OTHER PUBLICATIONS

Ross Laboratories: *Obstetrical Presentation and Position.* Columbus, Ohio, 1958.

Ross Laboratories: *Phenomena of Normal Labor.* Columbus, Ohio, 1964.

NOTES

Guide 10

ASSESSMENT OF DAVID WONDER

PART I. DAVID'S ASSESSMENT

You will be responsible for the initial nursing assessment of David Wonder after he is transferred to the nursery.

1. What are the reasons for performing a newborn nursing assessment?

2. Why is it important for you to know his prenatal and natal history when doing an assessment?

3. What types of information from the prenatal and natal history are significant in terms of the assessment?

4. Why is it necessary to assess David on more than one occasion?

5. You begin the assessment by observing David's general characteristics.

   a. State the average length of a newborn infant.

   b. State the usual weight range of newborn infants.

6. Next you observe the general characteristics of David's skin.

   a. State the usual expectations in relation to each of the characteristics listed below. Define any terms with which you are unfamiliar.

      1) Color (include expected changes when David cries)

      2) Desquamation

      3) Lanugo

      4) Vernix caseosa

5) Rashes (describe rashes of newborn; state when they usually occur)

6) Birth marks: hemangiomas

telangectasis

7) Bruises

8) Mottling

9) Milia

b. The following alterations may be seen. State the significance of each.

1) Color: jaundice

cyanosis

pallor

2) Impetigo

c. Nonwhite infants may have mongolian spots. What are these?

d. Describe the degree of development of David's sense of touch.

7. a. State the motor activity you would expect while David is:

1) Asleep

2) Awake

b. Describe the muscle tone of a normal newborn infant.

c. What position do newborn infants usually assume? Why?

d. 1) What changes in David's motor activity would indicate tetany?

2) What generally causes tetany in newborn infants?

3) How is it treated?

8. David has all of the reflexes listed on the next page. For each reflex:

a. Give a brief description of it.

b. State how you would test for it.

c. When appropriate, state the age at which it normally disappears.

d. State the significance of its absence or persistence.

REFLEX	*DESCRIPTION*	*HOW TESTED*	*AGE OF DISAPPEARANCE*	*SIGNIFICANCE OF ABSENCE OR PERSISTENCE*
Tonic neck				
Moro				
Grasp				
Plantar (foot)				
Babinski				
Step (Dance)				
Sucking				
Swallowing				

REFLEX	*DESCRIPTION*	*HOW TESTED*	*AGE OF DISAPPEARANCE*	*SIGNIFICANCE OF ABSENCE OR PERSISTENCE*
Rooting				
Swimming				

9. While observing David's head, you note an overriding of the sutures and some molding. Why do these occur?

10. a. What observations should be made in relation to David's anterior and posterior fontanels?

    b. What would a depressed fontanel indicate?

    c. What would a bulging or tense fontanel indicate?

    d. When does each fontanel usually close?

11. David does not have a cephalhematoma or craniotabes, but he does have caput succedaneum. Describe the following and state why they occur.

    a. Caput succedaneum

    b. Cephalhematoma

    c. Craniotabes

12. Intracranial hemorrhage is a possibility during delivery.

    a. Why does intracranial hemorrhage occur?

    b. What observations would indicate intracranial hemorrhage?

13. You will be observing David's ears.

    a. What observations will you make in relation to the characteristics of his ears?

    b. Describe the degree of development of David's hearing.

    c. How can his hearing be tested while he is in the nursery?

14. Describe the degree of development of David's sense of:

    a. Taste

    b. Smell

15. David's face appears to be symmetrical. What might asymmetry of the face indicate?

16. You observe David's eyes. You note their deep blue color and uncoordinated movements.

    a. How can you open David's eyes or have him open them?

b. If David's eyes change color, approximately when will this happen?

c. What is transient strabismus? Why is it common in newborn infants such as David?

d. David has a subconjunctival hemorrhage in his right eye.

1) What is a subconjunctival hemorrhage?

2) Why does it occur?

3) When will it disappear?

e. Describe the degree of development of David's vision. How can this be tested?

f. 1) When will David begin to have tears when he cries?

2) What would tearing of the eyes of a newborn indicate?

17. While inspecting David's mouth, you might note Epstein's pearls. What are these?

18. You will be observing David for cleft lip, cleft palate, thrush, and evidence of esophageal atresia and/or tracheoesophageal fistula.

    a. Briefly describe each of these conditions.

    b. State the observations you would make to detect it.

    c. Briefly state how it is treated.

        1) Cleft lip and palate

        2) Esophageal atresia and/or tracheoesophageal fistula

        3) Thrush

19. The circumference of David's head is 34.5 cm and the circumference of his chest is 33.5 cm.

    a. What is the average head and chest circumference of newborn infants?

    b. Are David's measurements within the average range?

    c. What should be the relationship between his head and chest size?

    d. What are the possible meanings of a discrepancy between head and chest circumference?

20. You observe David's neck.

    a. Compare the development of the neck of a newborn infant with that of an adult.

    b. Describe and state the observations that would indicate if David had:

        1) A hematoma of the sternocleidomastoid muscle

        2) Torticollis

21. a. Describe the cry of a normal newborn infant.

    b. Describe the abnormal cries of infants and their significance.

22. David's breasts are engorged.

    a. Why does this occur in newborn infants?

    b. What is "witch's milk"?

23. State the expected characteristics of David's apical heart beat.

24. State the expected characteristics of David's respirations.

25. a. How would you recognize abdominal distention in David?

    b. What might abdominal distention indicate?

26. a. Describe the expected changes in David's umbilical cord from birth until it separates from the infant.

    b. What changes would indicate an infected cord?

27. Occasionally these anomalies will be noted when inspecting an infant's abdomen. Briefly describe each.

    a. Exstrophy of the bladder

    b. Umbilical hernia

    c. Omphalocele

28. There is symmetry of size and movement of David's extremities. It is necessary to observe him for the deviations listed below. For each of these deviations:

    a. Briefly describe it.

    b. State the observations you would make to detect its presence or absence.

1) Brachial palsy

2) Fractured clavicle

3) Congenital dislocated hip

4) Syndactyly or polydactyly

5) Clubfoot

29. When you remove David's diaper you note that his urine appears pinkish. Why does this occur?

30. While observing David's genitalia, you will be looking for the following conditions. Briefly describe each.

a. Phimosis

b. Hypospadias

c. Epispadias

d. Undescended testes

e. Hydrocele

f. Smegma

31. If you were caring for a female infant, you would be observing her genitalia. Briefly describe the following:

a. Vaginal tag

b. Pseudomenstruation

c. Smegma

32. You will be observing David for an imperforate anus and meconium ileus. For each of these conditions:

a. Briefly describe it.

b. State the observations you would make which might indicate its presence.

1) Imperforate anus

2) Meconium ileus

33. When inspecting David's back, you will be observing for a pilonidal sinus or spina bifida. Briefly describe these deviations.

a. Pilonidal sinus

b. Spina bifida

PART II. GUIDE FOR ASSESSMENT OF NEWBORN INFANT

OBSERVATIONS	*POSSIBLE DEVIATIONS*
A. Prenatal and natal history	Complications of pregnancy, labor and delivery
B. General characteristics (infant lying supine)	
1. Skin:	
color	cyanosis
desquamation	jaundice
lanugo	erythroblastosis fetalis
vernix caseosa	impetigo
rashes	
birth marks	
bruises	
mottling	
tactile sense	
2. General body proportions	
head to body	prematurity
head circumference to chest circumference	hydrocephalus
length	microcephalus
weight	
3. Behavior	
motor activity	tetany
awake	
asleep	
position	
muscle tone	
4. Reflexes	
tonic neck	torticollis
Moro	fractured clavicle
step (dance) if held upright	brachial palsy
	CNS disturbances
C. Head	
craniotabes	cephalhematoma
caput succedaneum	hydrocephalus
ears:	microcephalus
position	craniosynostosis
formation	
hearing	
fontanels:	
anterior	
posterior	
circumference	
molding	
D. Face	
symmetry	facial paralysis
milia	ophthalmia neonatorum
eyes:	chemical conjunctivitis
blink	thrush
color	cleft lip
strabismus	cleft palate

OBSERVATIONS	*POSSIBLE DEVIATIONS*
reaction to light	esophageal atresia;
subconjunctival hemorrhage	tracheo-esophageal fistula
rooting reflex	
mouth:	
mouthing	
sucking pads	
sucking reflex	
Epstein's pearls	
retrusion tongue reflex	
E. Cry: character	brain damage
F. Neck: short	torticollis
	hematoma of sterno-cleidomastoid muscle
G. Chest	
respirations (rate, character)	respiratory distress
heart (rate, rhythm)	fractured clavicle
breast engorgement	
circumference	
H. Extremities	
symmetry of size and movement	brachial palsy
peripheral circulation	syndactyly
hands and feet:	polydactyly
grasp reflex	congenital dislocated hip
Babinski reflex	clubfoot
number of fingers and toes	
I. Abdomen	
shape	distention
symmetry	bleeding of cord
umbilical cord: number of vessels	omphalocele
	exstrophy of bladder
	infection of cord (omphalitis)
J. Genitalia	
edema	hypospadias
vaginal discharge	epispadias
vaginal tag	undescended testes
testes	hydrocele
K. Characteristics of infant when *prone*	
1. Neck:	
ability to support head	
2. Back:	spina bifida
mongolian spots	occulta
characteristics	meningocele
	myelomeningocele
3. Rectum:	
temperature	pilonidal sinus
stools	imperforate anus
	meconium ileus
4. Extremities:	
gluteal and thigh folds	congenital dislocated hip
swimming reflex	

REFERENCES

BOOKS

Blake, F. C., et al.: *Nursing Care of Children.* 8th Ed. Philadelphia, J. B. Lippincott Company, 1970.

Fitzpatrick, E., et al.: *Maternity Nursing.* 11th Ed. Philadelphia, J. B. Lippincott Company, 1966.

James, L. S.: "The Importance of Observations of the Newborn Infant at Birth." In Lytle, N. A., *Maternal Health Nursing,* pp. 97-107. Dubuque, Iowa, William C. Brown Company, Inc., 1967.

Marlow, D. R.: *Textbook of Pediatric Nursing.* 3rd Ed. Philadelphia, W. B. Saunders Company, 1969.

Wiedenbach, E.: *Family-Centered Maternity Nursing.* 2nd Ed. New York, G. P. Putnam's Sons, 1967.

JOURNAL ARTICLES

Battaglia, F. C.: "Recent Advances in Medicine for Newborn Infants." *Journal of Pediatrics,* 71:748, November 1967. (Association of obstetric complications with neonatal problems; treatment of idiopathic respiratory distress syndrome; intrauterine growth retardation; neonatal metabolic complications.)

Burnes, C. A.: "Patricia." *American Journal of Nursing,* 67:2576, December 1967. (Characteristics of a newborn infant.)

Fink, H. W.: "The Newborn at First Glance." *Hospital Topics,* 44:99, March 1966. (Observations of newborn; normal and abnormal characteristics.)

Green, M., and Richmond, J. B.: *Pediatric Diagnosis.* 2nd Ed., pp. 176-180. Philadelphia, W. B. Saunders Company, 1962. (Reflexes of newborn infant.)

Hervada, A. R.: "Nursery Evaluation of the Newborn." *American Journal of Nursing,* 67:1669, August 1967. (Significance of prenatal and natal history; Apgar score; characteristics and behavior of newborn.)

Jones, J. A.: "Examining the Newborn's Eyes: A Satisfactory Method." *Clinical Pediatrics,* 7:124, February 1968. (Illustrates method with two cotton-tipped applicators.)

Prystowsky, H.: "Intrauterine Growth and Development of the Baby." *Clinical Obstetrics and Gynecology,* 6:544, September 1963. (Fetal respiration, circulation, metabolic processes; neonatal blood counts; some abnormal neonatal conditions.)

Ravitch, M. M., and Rowe, M. I.: "Surgical Emergencies in the Neonate." *American Journal of Obstetrics and Gynecology,* 103:1034, April 1, 1969.

Reddell, R.: "Should Your Hospital Test Newborns' Hearing?" *Hospital Practice,* 5:107, February 1970. (Hearing tests for newborn infants.)

Shipe, D., et al.: "Neonatal Apgar Ratings as Related to Intelligence and Behavior in Preschool Children." *Child Development,* 39:861, September 1968. (Comparison of children with Apgar score below and above 5.)

OTHER PUBLICATIONS

Haynes, U.: *A Developmental Approach to Casefinding.* Washington, D.C., U.S. Department of Health, Education and Welfare, Children's Bureau Publication Number 449, 1967. (Perinatal mortality; appraisal of infants and young children.)

Mead Johnson Laboratories: *The Skin.* Evansville, Indiana, 1968.

Mead Johnson Laboratories: *The Head.* Evansville, Indiana, 1967.

Mead Johnson Laboratories: *The Eyes.* Evansville, Indiana, 1968.

Mead Johnson Laboratories: *Birthmarks.* Evansville, Indiana, 1968.

Mead Johnson Laboratories: *The Mouth.* Evansville, Indiana, 1969.

Mead Johnson Laboratories: *The External Ear.* Evansville, Indiana, 1970.

Public Health Service: *Spinal Birth Defects.* Washington, D.C., U.S. Department of Health, Education and Welfare.

Ross Laboratories: *Common Variations in the Neonate.* Columbus, Ohio, 1961.

NOTES

Guide 11

AMY WONDER'S POSTPARTUM

PART I. AMY WONDER'S FIRST HOUR POSTPARTUM

Following delivery of her baby, Amy was moved to the recovery room in another area of the delivery suite.

1. What is the rationale for keeping Amy in a recovery room for a period of time after delivery rather than sending her back to her room immediately?

2. Why is the first hour following delivery (also referred to as the fourth stage of labor) a critical time for Amy?

Thirty minutes after Amy's delivery, you note the following:

fundus: firm, at level of umbilicus, displaced to right side
lochia: profuse, rubra, two pads saturated within 15 minutes

3. a. What is the fundus?

   1) Where should the fundus be located at this time?

   2) What will you do if Amy's fundus becomes soft and boggy?

3) What medications are frequently given to help the uterus maintain a contracted state?

4) How frequently should you check Amy's fundus during the first hour postpartum? Why?

5) What is the probable cause of Amy's fundus being displaced to one side? What nursing intervention is indicated?

b. What is lochia?

1) Describe the expected characteristics of Amy's lochia during the first hour postpartum.

2) How frequently should the lochia be checked during this time? Why?

4. Amy's blood pressure is 120/68, pulse 76 and respirations 20. What is the rationale for taking Amy's blood pressure, pulse and respirations following delivery?

5. Amy complains of feeling chilled and you notice she is shaking.

   a. What are the possible causes of a "chill" at this time?

   b. What nursing intervention is indicated?

6. Harold comes to the recovery room with Amy. What is your role in supporting Harold at this time?

PART II. AMY WONDER'S CARE

It is necessary for you to understand the changes which are taking place as you care for Amy during her postpartal period. Amy also needs to know what changes she can expect.

7. During Amy's puerperium, involution is taking place.

a. Define puerperium.

b. What is the process of involution?

8. Amy's uterus will undergo changes during the puerperium.

a. State the rate of change in the height of the fundus during Amy's postpartal period which indicates that involution is occurring satisfactorily.

b. State the changes in Amy's lochia (color, consistency, amount, odor) which would indicate that involution is occurring satisfactorily.

c. State the changes which occur in the cervix during the puerperium.

9. You observe that Amy is perspiring profusely. Why does this occur?

10. Amy wants to know if her "stretch marks" will disappear. What changes in Amy's abdominal wall can be expected during this period?

11. Amy's obstetrician has ordered Empirin compound with codeine phosphate no. 3 PRN for discomfort.

   a. What is the action of this medication?

   b. What are the implications for nursing care when administering this medication?

12. Amy's obstetrician wants her to be out of bed for a few minutes six hours following delivery.

   a. What are the advantages of early ambulation following delivery?

   b. State the nurse's responsibilities in assisting Amy the first time she gets out of bed.

c. Amy states that there is an increase in lochia when she first gets up. What is the significance of this increased lochia?

13. Amy wants to be weighed when she gets up to take her shower the morning following delivery. She finds she has lost 12 pounds. She comments that the baby only weighed 7½ pounds. How will you explain the other 4½ pound weight loss to Amy?

14. You are with Amy when she gets ready for her shower.

 a. What are the criteria for deciding whether the patient should have a tub bath or shower?

 b. Differentiate between a tub bath and sitz bath.

 c. State the safety measures to be considered by the nurse when Amy takes her first shower.

 d. State the knowledge Amy needs concerning the care of her breasts when she showers.

15. You will be teaching Amy how to do her own perineal care.

a. Why is it necessary for Amy to know proper perineal care?

b. State the scientific principles you will teach Amy to apply when she gives herself perineal care.

16. Amy has difficulty voiding following delivery.

a. Why does difficulty in voiding frequently occur during the puerperium?

b. What are the consequences if Amy is unable to void?

c. State the observations you will make which are indicative of a full bladder.

d. State several nursing measures which may encourage Amy to void.

e. State the principles you will follow if it becomes necessary to catheterize Amy.

17. Amy complains of discomfort from her episiotomy sutures on the second postpartum day. You note the area is slightly edematous but not red.

a. What is the significance of this observation?

b. State several nursing measures which will be helpful in relieving Amy's discomfort.

c. State the purpose of each of the measures identified above.

18. The afternoon of her first postpartal day, you find Amy in the bathroom; she is perspiring and says she "feels faint." She tells you she is trying to have a bowel movement.

a. What are the physiological reasons that she might perspire and feel faint?

b. What will you do?

19. a. What exercises might Amy be taught during the puerperium?

b. State the purposes of each of these exercises.

REFERENCES

BOOKS

Bergersen, B. S., and Krug, E. E.: *Pharmacology in Nursing.* 11th Ed. St. Louis, The C. V. Mosby Company, 1969.

Bryant, R. D., and Overland, A. E.: *Woodward and Gardner's Obstetric Management and Nursing.* 7th Ed. Philadelphia, F. A. Davis Company, 1964.

Eastman, N. J., and Hellman, L. M.: *Williams Obstetrics.* 12th Ed., pp. 494-510. New York, Appleton-Century-Crofts, Inc., 1961.

Fitzpatrick, E., et al.: *Maternity Nursing.* 11th Ed. Philadelphia, J. B. Lippincott Company, 1966.

Rodman, M. J., and Smith, D. W.: *Pharmacology and Drug Therapy in Nursing.* Philadelphia, J. B. Lippincott Company, 1968.

Wiedenbach, E.: *Family-Centered Maternity Care.* 2nd Ed. New York, G. P. Putnam's Sons, 1967.

Ziegel, E., and Van Blarcom, C. C.: *Obstetric Nursing.* 5th Ed., pp. 417-483. New York, The Macmillan Company, 1965.

JOURNAL ARTICLES

Beck, P., et al.: "Insertion of an Intrauterine Contraceptive Device at Time of Delivery: A Preliminary Study." *Ob/Gyn Digest,* 10:42, August 1968.

Booker, D. E., et al.: "Control of Postpartum Breast Engorgement with Oral Contraceptives." *American Journal of Obstetrics and Gynecology,* 108:240, September 15, 1970.

Cibils, L. A., and Hendricks, C. H.: "Uterine Contractility on the First Day of the Puerperium." *American Journal of Obstetrics and Gynecology,* 103:238, January 15, 1969.

Frank, R., et al.: "Oral Contraceptives Started Early in the Puerperium." *American Journal of Obstetrics and Gynecology,* 103:112, January 1, 1969.

Hendrick, W.: "An Elderly Primigravida Takes a 'Refresher Course' in Obstetrics." *American Journal of Nursing,* 70:787, April 1970. (Compares her pregnancy with textbook picture; describes care received; states that the care not received was appalling.)

Larsen, V. L.: "Stresses of the Childbearing Year." *American Journal of Public Health,* 56:32, January 1966. (Stresses during pregnancy, labor and delivery; postpartum and first three months at home.)

McCain, F. R.: "Nursing by Assessment – Not Intuition." *American Journal of Nursing,* 65:82, April 1965.

Nedbor, P., and Averette, H.: "Hospital Institutes Program for Self Perineal Care." *Hospital Topics,* 46:81, May 1968.

Rubin, R.: "Puerperal Change." *Nursing Outlook,* 9:753, December 1961. (Anatomical, physiological and psychological changes, "taking-in" and "taking-hold.")

Smith, R. A., and Juan, M., Sr.: "Postpartum Tub Bath." *American Journal of Nursing,* 64:135, September 1964.

Woessner, J. F.: "Postpartum Involution of the Uterus Connective Tissue Framework." *Ob/Gyn Digest,* 10:44, July 1968.

Yunek, M. J.: "Postpartum Care Is More than a Routine." *Nursing Outlook,* 17:50, June 1969.

OTHER PUBLICATIONS

Rose, P. A.: "Identification and Application of Psychiatric Principles in the Nursing Care of Maternity Patients." *Phases in Human Development: Relevance in Nursing,* pp. 14-36. ANA 1962 Clinical Sessions, 10 Columbus Circle, New York. (Detailed analysis of a nurse's interaction with a 19-year-old primipara during labor, delivery and postpartum. Some interaction with husband.)

NOTES

Guide 12

THE WONDERS: A FAMILY OF THREE

PART I. AMY, DAVID AND HAROLD

Amy and Harold had decided that Amy would breast feed their baby. Today (her second postpartal day), she tells you this may have been the wrong decision, because the baby does not seem to be getting enough milk. She says that her breasts are small and she is sure this is the problem. There are tears in her eyes when she adds, "I wanted so badly to breast feed him."

1. In order to discuss this with Amy, you must have accurate knowledge of the process of lactation.

   a. Define lactation.

   b. Name the hormone which initiates lactation.

   c. State the structure responsible for the production of milk.

   d. State the structures which secrete milk.

e. What is the let-down reflex (milk-ejection reflex, draught reflex)?

1) What causes the occurrence of the let-down reflex?

2) What inhibits the let-down reflex?

3) When can Amy anticipate the let-down reflex will occur?

f. Before Amy's milk "comes in," her breasts contain colostrum. What is colostrum?

g. Amy's breasts will become engorged.

1) When will this occur?

2) Why does breast engorgement occur?

3) What nursing measures can be taken to relieve Amy's discomfort while her breasts are engorged?

h. If Amy was not going to breast feed her baby, what medications might be ordered to inhibit lactation?

i. What suggestions will you give Amy to help her:

1) Avoid cracked nipples

2) Care for cracked nipples if this condition occurs

2. State the knowledge and skills Amy will need as she learns to breast feed her infant in relation to:

a. Sucking and reflex behavior of infants

b. Positioning herself and infant

c. Length of nursing time

d. Schedule of feeding

e. Supplemental (complemental) feedings

f. Effects of drugs and diet on breast milk

3. What nursing intervention is indicated in relation to Amy's concern about her decision to breast feed her infant?

4. Amy and Harold have decided to name their son David Newman Wonder. His birth certificate will be completed and registered with the local registrar.

    a. What information will be available on David's birth certificate?

    b. Why is it necessary to register all births?

    c. Who is responsible for registering David's birth?

5. Amy and her son have a rooming-in arrangment.

    a. What is rooming-in?

    b. What are the advantages of rooming-in to:

        1) Amy (mother)

        2) Harold (father)

3) David (infant)

4) The nurse

c. What are the possible disadvantages of rooming-in to:

1) Amy

2) Harold

3) David

4) The nurse

6. "Taking-in" and "taking-hold" are two phases which have been identified by Reva Rubin as occurring during the puerperium. State the behaviors which will probably be exhibited by Amy during each phase.

   a. "Taking-in" phase

   b. "Taking-hold" phase

7. During Amy's puerperium, you observe behaviors which are indicative of developing motherliness.

   a. What is motherliness?

   b. What factors contribute to the attainment of motherliness?

   c. When does motherliness usually begin to develop?

d. Is motherliness achieved at the same rate by all mothers? Explain your answer.

e. How can the nurse assist Amy in achieving optimal attainment of motherliness?

8. On the third postpartum day, you note that Amy says very little, does not smile and cries easily. This behavior is indicative of the "postpartum blues."

   a. What causes postpartum blues?

   b. What support can you give Amy during this period?

c. What support can you give Harold during this period?

d. What support can Harold give Amy during this time?

9. Harold visits Amy and David daily. During this time he usually holds David as he talks with his wife. He states that he "just can't believe" he is a father.

   a. What is fatherliness?

   b. How does fatherliness develop?

PART II. AMY'S PREPARATION FOR HOME

Since Amy and David have a rooming-in arrangement, you have many opportunities to guide Amy in planning for the baby's care when she returns home. Amy has attended prenatal classes but needs reinforcement concerning her care and the baby's care.

10. You will be teaching Amy about her own care as well as the care of her baby.

    a. What behaviors of Amy will indicate she is ready to learn?

    b. How will you determine how much she can absorb at one time?

11. Amy has many questions about the baby's behavior, such as hiccoughing, yawning, quivering of the chin. State the knowledge Amy needs about each of these infant behaviors.

12. Amy is concerned about the baby's appearance. Identify at least six characteristics of a newborn infant which might be interpreted as abnormal by his mother and state what you would tell Amy about each.

13. Amy is concerned she will not know what to do when David cries at home. State the knowledge which will be helpful to Amy in interpreting David's crying.

14. Amy will be preparing sterile water and supplemental feedings for David.

    a. State the principles of formula preparation which Amy needs to understand.

    b. Amy asks, "Which is the best method for preparing the formula?" State the knowledge you need about formula preparation in order to answer Amy's question.

    c. What additional information from Amy would be useful in answering this question?

15. Amy will be bathing David in the sink or in a small plastic tub at home.

a. State the principles of bathing a baby you will teach Amy.

b. State the safety measures you want to be certain Amy understands in relation to bathing her infant.

16. Identify the other areas related to David's care in which education is needed before Amy is discharged. Briefly state the information Amy needs about each of these areas.

17. Amy also needs instruction concerning her own care after she gets home. State the information Amy needs related to her:

    a. Breasts

    b. Perineum

    c. Diet (she is breast feeding)

    d. Rest

e. Activity

REFERENCES

BOOKS

Anthony, E. J., and Benedek, T. (Eds.): *Parenthood – Its Psychology and Psychopathology.* Boston, Little, Brown and Company, 1970.

Callon, H.: "Consultation – a Tool for Helping Mothers." In Bergersen, B. S., et al. (Eds.): *Current Concepts in Clinical Nursing.* Vol. 2, Chapter 24. St. Louis, The C. V. Mosby Company, 1969. (Nurse's role; self-understanding; understanding mothers and families; objectives of consultation; methods of meeting objectives.)

Clark, A. L.: *Leadership Technique in Expectant Parent Education.* New York, Springer Publishing Company, Inc., 1962.

La Leche League International: *The Womanly Art of Breastfeeding.* Franklin Park, Illinois, La Leche League International, 1963.

Lally, A. T.: "Perspectives on Rooming-in." In Bergersen, B. S., et al. (Eds.): *Current Concepts in Clinical Nursing.* Vol. 2, Chapter 28. St. Louis, The C. V. Mosby Company, 1969. (Advantages of rooming-in; how it can be managed under various circumstances; nurse's role.)

Lidz, T.: *The Person: His Development Throughout the Life Cycle,* pp. 93-116. New York, Basic Books, Inc., 1968.

Netter, F. H.: *The Ciba Collection of Medical Illustrations.* Vol. 2. *Reproductive System.* New York, Ciba Corporation, 1965.

Newton, M., and Newton, N.: "The Normal Course and Management of Lactation." In Lytle, N. A.: *Maternal Health Nursing,* pp. 108-126. Dubuque, Iowa, William C. Brown Company, Inc., 1967.

Nordmark, M. T., and Rohweder, A. W.: *Scientific Foundations of Nursing.* 2nd Ed., pp. 134-136. Philadelphia, J. B. Lippincott Company, 1967. (Sleep and rest.)

Orlando, I. J.: *The Dynamic Nurse-Patient Relationship.* New York, G. P. Putnam's Sons, 1961.

Schaefer, G., and Zisowitz, M. L.: *The Expectant Father.* New York, Simon and Schuster, 1964.

Wiedenbach, E.: *Family-Centered Maternity Care.* 2nd Ed. New York, G. P. Putnam's Sons, 1967.

Williams, S. R.: *Nutrition and Diet Therapy.* St. Louis, The C. V. Mosby Company, 1969.

JOURNAL ARTICLES

Applebaum, R. M.: "The Modern Management of Successful Breast Feeding." *Pediatric Clinics of North America,* 17:203, February 1970. (Prenatal, hospital and postpartal period; anatomy and physiology of lactation.)

Auerbach, A. B.: "Meeting the Needs of New Mothers." *Children,* 11:223, November-December 1964. (Includes feelings and fears of parents during pregnancy and puerperium; needs for education.)

Booker, D. E., et al.: "Control of Postpartum Breast Engorgement with Oral Contraceptives." *American Journal of Obstetrics and Gynecology,* 108:240, September 15, 1970.

Carroll, G. H.: "First Time Parents." *Child and Family,* 4:13, Spring 1965. (Development of motherliness and fatherliness.)

Clark, A. L.: "The Beginning Family." *American Journal of Nursing,* 66:802, April 1966. (The phases of establishment; childbearing and childrearing; postpartal needs. Teaching.)

Disbrow, M. A.: "Any Woman Who Really Wants to Nurse Her Baby Can Do So?" *Nursing Forum,* 2(3):39, 1963. (Mothers' reactions to breast feeding; implications for nursing.)

Dyal, L., and Kahrl, J.: "When Mothers Breast Feed." *American Journal of Nursing,* 67:2555, December 1967. (Students' feelings concerning mothers who are breast feeding and suggestions for helping those mothers.)

"Economy in Nutrition and Feeding of Infants." *American Journal of Public Health,* 56:1756, October 1966. (Infant feeding in the family setting; nutritional status of infants; meeting infants' nutritional needs; costs.)

Eppirk, H.: "An Experiment to Determine a Basis for Nursing Decisions in Regard to Time of Initiation of Breastfeeding." *Nursing Research,* 18:292, July-August 1969. (A study of two groups of babies introduced to breast feeding.)

Gordon, R. E., et al.: "Factors in Postpartum Emotional Adjustment." *Obstetrics and Gynecology,* 25:158, February 1967.

Iffrig, M. C., Sr.: "Nursing Care and Success in Breast Feeding." *Nursing Clinics of North America,* 3:345, June 1968. (Specific prenatal preparation; breast feeding and alternate massage.)

Klaus, M. H., et al.: "Human Maternal Behavior at the First Contact with Her Young." *Pediatrics,* 46:187, August 1970. (Mothers' initial contact with their normal newborn infants and with premature infants in Isolettes.)

Larsen, V. L.: "Stresses of the Childbearing Year." *American Journal of Public Health,* 56:32, January 1966.

Leifer, G.: "Rooming-in Despite Postpartal Complications." *American Journal of Nursing,* 67:2114, October 1967. (Comprehensive report of postpartal rooming-in experience for mother with thrombophlebitis; includes nursing care plan.)

Lichter, J. M.: "Infection Control in Maternity Units." *Nursing Outlook,* 12:32, August 1964. (Rooming-in units; methods of control.)

Newton, M.: "Nine Questions Mothers May Ask about Breast-Feeding." *Consultant,* 7:27, February 1967. (What may be behind the questions; suggested responses; recommended books on breast feeding for mothers.)

Newton, N., and Newton, M.: "Mothers' Reactions to Their Newborn Babies." *Journal of the American Medical Association,* 181:206, July 21, 1962. (Factors which may influence reactions; behavior of rejecting and accepting mothers; implications.)

Rubin, R.: "Basic Maternal Behavior." *Nursing Outlook,* 9:683, November 1961. (Mothers' behavior toward newborn; identification process.)

Rubin, R.: "Food and Feeding." *Nursing Forum,* 6:195, Spring 1967. (Interpersonal relationships.)

Rubin, R.: "Maternal Touch," *Nursing Outlook,* 11:828, November 1963. (Development of maternal touch; the nurse's touch.)

Rubin, R.: "Puerperal Change." *Nursing Outlook,* 9:753, December 1961. (Anatomical, physiological and psychological changes; "taking-in" and "taking-hold.")

"A Salute to La Leche League International." *The Journal of Pediatrics,* 73:161, July 1968.

Schmitt, M. H.: "Superiority of Breast-Feeding: Fact or Fancy?" *American Journal of Nursing,* 70:1488, July 1970. (Review of literature for empirical evidence of values of breast feeding.)

Shainess, N.: "Motherhood: A Tempering Experience." *Child and Family,* 4:3, Spring 1965. (Development of maternal attitude – mothering.)

Smith, B. B.: "Breast Feeding: Facts and Fallacies." *Today's Health,* 44:37, February 1966.

Vaughan, V. C.: "A Study of Techniques of Preparation of Formulas for Infant Feeding." *Journal of Pediatrics,* 61:547, October 1962. (Prevalent Practices in formula preparation; implications.)

Wessel, M. A.: "Maternal and Child Nursing – as a Pediatrician Sees it." *Nursing Outlook,* 11:207, March 1963.

Weston, J. L.: "Initiating Referrals: A Health Department Approach." *American Journal of Nursing,* 67:332, February 1967. (Informal sessions on the maternity ward as the initial public health center to provide continuity of care for families.)

Yunek, M. J.: "Postpartum Care Is More than a Routine." *Nursing Outlook,* 17:50, June 1969.

OTHER PUBLICATIONS

Anderson, E. H.: "A Study of Postpartum Depression: Implications for Nursing." *Designs for Nurse-Patient Interaction,* pp. 5-13. ANA 1964 Clinical Sessions, 10 Columbus Circle, New York. (Study of 38 primiparas, incidence and nature of depression, motives of postpartum depression, clues to depression; suggestions for nursing.)

Branin, V. A.: "A Study of Problems Encountered by Twenty-Six Nursing Mothers Following Hospital Discharge." *Evaluation of Nursing Intervention,* pp. 13-18. ANA 1964 Clinical Sessions, 10 Columbus Circle, New York. (Seminar for nursing mothers; their experiences and problems; implications for nursing assistance.)

Children's Bureau: *Costs of Formulas for Babies Differ.* Washington, D.C., U.S. Government Printing Office, U.S. Department of Health, Education and Welfare, 1968.

Children's Bureau: *Evaporated Milk – a Good Formula for Babies: A Day's Supply that Won't Sour.* Washington, D.C., U.S. Government Printing Office, U.S. Department of Health, Education and Welfare, 1969.

Children's Bureau: *Evaporated Milk – a Good Formula for Babies: Single Bottle Method.* U.S. Government Printing Office, U.S. Department of Health, Education and Welfare, 1969.

Children's Bureau: *Infant Care.* U.S. Government Printing Office, U.S.Department of Health, Education and Welfare, 1963.

Disbrow, M. A.: "Nursing Intervention as a Factor in Successful Breast Feeding." *Evaluation of Nursing Intervention,* pp. 5-12. ANA 1964 Clinical Sessions, 10 Columbus Circle, New York. (Problems encountered in breast feeding; implications for nursing intervention.)

Haire, D.: *Instructions for Nursing Your Baby.* New Jersey, International Childbirth Education Association, 1969.

International Childbirth Education Association: "Check List for Counseling Breast-Feeding Mothers." Hillside, New Jersey. (Possible causes of mothers' concerns, such as sore nipples, insufficient milk.)

La Leche League International, Inc.: *Breastfeeding Your Baby.* Franklin Park, Illinois, 1968.
La Leche League International, Inc.: *When You Breast Feed Your Baby.* Franklin Park, Illinois, 1966.
Mead Johnson and Company: *Breast Feeding Your Baby.* Evansville, Indiana, 1968.
Ross Laboratories: "Anticipatory Guidance." *Currents in Public Health,* Vol. 3, Number 4, April 1963.
Ross Laboratories: *Breast Feeding Your Baby.* Columbus, Ohio, 1969.
Ross Laboratories: *The Mammary Glands and Breast Feeding.* Columbus, Ohio, 1962.
William S. Merrell Company: *Lactation. A Programmed Review.* Cincinnati, Ohio, 1967.

NOTES

Guide 13

THE SWEETS' BABY IS STILLBORN

PART I. SUSAN SWEET'S ANTEPARTAL CARE

You visit Susan Sweet in her home because she has failed to keep her last two clinic appointments. She is a 34-year-old gravida 4 para 2 who has had diabetes for the past 5 years, "ever since I had my first kid." She is now 4½ months pregnant and knows she "should have come to clinic sooner, but just couldn't get away from the house." Her first and only clinic visit was one month ago. At that time, her regular and NPH insulin dosage was adjusted and she was to return in two weeks. Susan has had one previous spontaneous abortion and is "praying everything will be O.K. this time."

1. What is the meaning of gravida 4 para 2?

2. Susan Sweet's pregnancy is considered high risk.

   a. Why is her pregnancy classified as high risk?

   b. What implications does this have for nursing?

3. Susan has diabetes, which causes additional physiological stress on her and her unborn baby. State the:

   a. Physiological relationship between Susan's pregnancy and diabetes

   b. Effect the diabetes may have on her baby

   c. Usual medical management of diabetes during pregnancy

   d. Knowledge Susan should have about the management of her pregnancy and diabetes

4. Susan has missed two scheduled clinic appointments because she "couldn't get out of the house."

   a. What knowledge about Susan would help you in assessing this statement?

   b. How can you assist Susan in receiving the medical and nursing care she needs?

5. Susan's last pregnancy ended with a spontaneous abortion.

   a. How does a spontaneous abortion differ from a therapeutic abortion?

   b. For each classification of abortion listed below:

      1) State the characteristics of each

      2) Indicate its medical management

      3) State the nurse's role in caring for a woman with that type of abortion

CLASSIFICATION	*CHARACTERISTICS*	*MEDICAL CARE*	*NURSING CARE*
Threatened			
Inevitable			
Incomplete			
Complete			
Missed			

c. What are the causes of spontaneous abortions?

d. What are habitual abortions?

e. 1) What are the usual indications for therapeutic abortions?

2) What are the current trends regarding laws in the United States related to therapeutic abortion?

f. 1) What is a criminal abortion?

2) Who usually performs criminal abortions?

3) What are the dangers when a criminal abortion is performed?

Susan's last pregnancy terminated in a spontaneous abortion.

6. She first became aware of the difficulty when she began to have vaginal bleeding. For each of the causes of bleeding listed below, state the:

   a. Trimester during which the condition usually occurs

   b. Possible causes of the condition

   c. Approximate amount of bleeding

   d. Characteristics of pain if pain is present

   e. Effects of the condition on the onset of labor

   f. Usual medical intervention

   g. Nursing intervention related to the medical intervention, anticipatory guidance and support of mother and family

	SPONTANEOUS ABORTION	*PLACENTA PREVIA*	*ABRUPTIO PLACENTA*
Trimester occurring			
Possible causes			
Bleeding			
Pain			

	SPONTANEOUS ABORTION	*PLACENTA PREVIA*	*ABRUPTIO PLACENTA*
Effects on labor onset			
Medical intervention			
Nursing intervention			

PART II. SUSAN SWEET'S LABOR AND DELIVERY

You are unable to hear any fetal heart tones when Susan arrives in the labor room. The obstetrician examines Susan and tells her that her baby is dead. Susan had been having mild irregular contractions prior to coming to the hospital. She says she does not recall any fetal activity today, "but there have been other days when the baby didn't move much." She is in her 37th week of gestation. Her husband, Steven, is in the waiting room.

7. What nursing support does Susan Sweet need at this time?

8. What factors will determine if Steven Sweet should be in the labor room with his wife?

9. How will the nursing management of Susan's labor compare with the management of a woman, such as Amy Wonder, whose labor is progressing satisfactorily?

10. Susan is medicated with meperidine hydrochloride (Demerol) and scopolamine hydrobromide to produce twilight sleep during the remainder of her labor. State the implications this has for her nursing care.

PART III. SUSAN SWEET'S POSTPARTAL EXPERIENCE

11. Susan has cried frequently, but said little since the delivery 15 hours ago. As you are with her, she makes a number of statements. For each of Susan's statements listed below state:

    a. What you think is being expressed even though it is not verbalized explicitly

    b. The nursing intervention which would be appropriate

        1) "What have I done to deserve this?"

        2) "I'm glad the baby was born dead instead of living a few weeks and then dying."

        3) "I know there must have been something wrong with the baby that they're not telling me about. Why won't they tell me?"

4) "My husband didn't want me to get pregnant anyway."

12. Susan saw her baby while she was still in the delivery room. Her husband saw the baby before she was taken from the delivery area. What are the pros and cons of the Sweets' seeing their stillborn baby?

13. Susan has cried frequently since the baby's birth and Steven has been unable to sleep or discuss the birth with anyone. They are grieving for the loss of their baby.

    a. Describe the process of grieving.

b. Identify the nurse's role in therapeutically supporting Susan and Steven Sweet during each phase of the grieving process.

c. State how your background and your feelings and attitudes about death, especially the death of an infant, affect the support you will be able to give the Sweets.

d. How can you become more aware of your feelings and gain support while you are coping with these feelings?

14. The Sweets have two boys at home, a five-year-old and a three-year-old. The boys have been prepared for the birth of this baby and were excited when Mrs. Sweet left for the hospital yesterday. What suggestions can you make to help the Sweets explain to their boys that there will be no baby to bring home?

15. Susan Sweet said she was glad the baby had not lived for a few weeks before dying. There are occasions when the death of a newborn infant can be anticipated because of abnormalities incompatible with life.

    a. What are the advantages and disadvantages to the parents of having contact with the infant under these circumstances?

    b. What factors will determine whether the parents have any contact with the infant who is not going to survive?

REFERENCES

BOOKS

Arnstein, H. S.: *What to Tell Your Child.* Indianapolis, The Bobbs-Merrill Company, Inc., 1962. (About death.)

Bergersen, B. S., and Krug, E. E.: *Pharmacology in Nursing.* 11th Ed. St. Louis, The C. V. Mosby Company, 1969.

Bryant, R. D., and Overland, A. E.: *Woodward and Gardner's Obstetric Management and Nursing.* 7th Ed. Philadelphia, F. A. Davis Company, 1964.

Eastman, N. J., and Hellman, L. M.: *Williams Obstetrics.* 12th Ed., pp. 525-560. New York, Appleton-Century-Crofts, Inc., 1961.

Fitzpatrick, E., et al.: *Maternity Nursing.* 11th Ed. Philadelphia, J. B. Lippincott Company, 1966.

Glaser, B. G., and Strauss, A. L.: *Awareness of Dying.* Chicago, Aldine Publishing Company, 1965.

Hall, R. E. (Ed.): *Abortion in a Changing World.* Vol. 1. New York, Columbia University Press, 1970.

Lee, N. H.: *The Search for an Abortionist.* Chicago, The University of Chicago Press, 1969.

Lerch, C.: *Maternity Nursing.* St. Louis, The C. V. Mosby Company, 1970.

Moriarity, D. M. (Ed.): *The Loss of Loved Ones.* Springfield, Illinois, Charles C Thomas, Publisher, 1967. (Effects of a death in the family on personality development.)

Nordmark, M. T., and Rohweder, A. W.: *Scientific Foundations of Nursing.* 2nd Ed. Philadelphia, J. B. Lippincott Company, 1967.

Orlando, I. J.: *The Dynamic Nurse-Patient Relationship.* New York, G. P. Putnam's Sons, 1961.

Rodman, M. J., and Smith, D. W.: *Pharmacology and Drug Therapy in Nursing.* Philadelphia, J. B. Lippincott Company, 1968.

Shnider, S. M. (Ed.): *Obstetrical Anesthesia – Current Concepts and Practice.* Baltimore, The Williams and Wilkins Company, 1970.

Williams, S. R.: *Nutrition and Diet Therapy.* St. Louis, The C. V. Mosby Company, 1969.

Ziegel, E., and Van Blarcom, C. C.: *Obstetric Nursing.* 5th Ed., pp. 149-197. New York, The Macmillan Company, 1965.

JOURNAL ARTICLES

Apgar, V., and Stickle, G.: "Birth Defects." *Journal of the American Medical Association,* 204:371, April 29, 1968. (Definition and taxonomy; fetal loss; prevalence.)

Bartsch, V.: "Standardization of Terminology, Reporting of Live Births, Fetal Deaths." *Hospital Topics,* 46:97, February 1968. (Birth certificate; fetal death certificate.)

Beck, M. B., et al.: "Abortion: A National Public and Mental Health Problem – Past, Present, and Proposed Research." *American Journal of Public Health,* 59:2131, December 1969. (Incidence; motivations for abortions; legislation.)

Brandt, M. B.: "Nutrition in Pregnancy." *Clinical Obstetrics and Gynecology,* 6:604, September 1963.

Bruce, S. J.: "Reactions of Nurses and Mothers to Stillbirths." *Nursing Outlook,* 10:88, February 1962. (Feelings of 25 graduate nurses and 25 mothers; guilt; acceptance of reality; grief.)

Buxton, C. L.: "One Doctor's Opinion of Abortion Laws." *American Journal of Nursing,* 68:1026, May 1968.

Caillouette, J. C.: "Septic Abortion: Pathology and Treatment." *American Journal of Nursing,* 66:1045, May 1966.

Conant, L. H.: "Give-and-Take in Home Visits." *American Journal of Nursing,* 65:117, July 1965. (Communication – verbal and non-verbal; patients' and nurses' reactions to home visits.)

Downs, F. S.: "Maternal Stress in Primigravidas as a Factor in the Production of Neonatal Pathology." *Nursing Science,* 2:348, October 1964. (Reviews causes of perinatal morbidity and mortality; report of research to investigate relationship to maternal stress and neonatal pathology.)

Dwyer, J. M.: "Transplantation Immunity and the Human Placenta." *American Journal of Nursing,* 68:1712, August, 1968. (Study of immune responses to tissue transplants from husbands as a possible cause for repeated abortions in some women.)

Engel, G.: "Grief and Grieving." *American Journal of Nursing,* 64:92, September 1964.

Fornseca, J. D.: "Induced Abortion, Nursing Attitudes and Action." *American Journal of Nursing,* 68:1022, May 1968.

Garnet, J. D.: "Pregnancy in Women with Diabetes." *American Journal of Nursing,* 69:1900, September 1969. (Overview of management; characteristics of newborn infant.)

Gold, E. M.: "Identification of the High Risk Fetus." *Clinical Obstetrics and Gynecology,* 11:1069, December 1968. (Assessment of infant mortality and morbidity; criteria for identifying high risk pregnancy and high risk infant; application of criteria.)

Goldstein, J.: "Exploring Attitudes that Affect Nursing Care." *Nursing Outlook,* 16:50, June 1968. (Attitudes of practical nursing students toward death and birth.)

Gray, J. W.: "Liaison Nurses Bridge the Care Gap." *Nursing Outlook,* 15:28, May 1967. (Nurses act as liaison for high risk maternity patients between clinic, hospital and community.)

Ingram, J. M.: "Changing Aspects of Abortion Law." *American Journal of Obstetrics and Gynecology,* 105:35, September 1, 1969.

Kallaus, J.: "The Child with Cleft Lip and Palate – the Mother in the Maternity Unit." *American Journal of Nursing,* 65:120, April 1965. (Reactions of mothers to deformed newborns – suggestions for nursing intervention.)

Larsen, V. L.: "Stresses of the Childbearing Year." *American Journal of Public Health,* 56:32, January 1966.

McKay, R. J., and Lucey, J. F.: "Neonatology." *The New England Journal of Medicine,* 270-1231, June 4, 1964. (Drugs; immunity; respiratory distress syndrome; infants of diabetic mothers; hypoglycemia.)

McKay, R. J., and Lucey, J. F.: "Neonatology." *The New England Journal of Medicine,* 270:1292, June 11, 1964. (Jaundice; twins; prematurity; aids to diagnosing neonatal disease.)

McLenahan, I. G.: "Helping the Mother Who Has no Baby to Take Home." *American Journal of Nursing,* 62:70, April 1962. (Consideration of grief and death for mother and nurse; implications for nursing.)

Marshall, M. H.: "Septic Abortion: Crisis Care." *American Journal of Nursing,* 66:1042, May 1966. (Overview of information regarding abortions and care during the crisis stage.)

Masco, J., Sr.: "This One Was Different." *American Journal of Nursing,* 67:1898, September 1967. (Experience during pregnancy, labor, delivery, and postpartal period of a woman who gave birth to a stillborn infant.)

Nesbitt, R. E. L., and Richard, A. H.: "High-Risk Obstetrics." *American Journal of Obstetrics and Gynecology,* 103:972, April 1, 1969.

"Reducing Infant Mortality: Suggested Approaches." *Journal of the American Medical Association,* 193:310, July 26, 1965. (Mortality rates; definitions of rates; factors influencing mortality; high risk pregnancy; care needed.)

"The Right to Abortion: A Psychiatric View." *Group for the Advancement of Psychiatry.* Vol. 7, Number 75, October 1969.

Robischon, P.: "The Challenge of Crisis Theory for Nursing." *Nursing Outlook,* 15:28, July 1967. (Types of crises – developmental and situational; includes birth of an atypical child; parenthood; general principles applicable to crisis intervention.)

Rose, P. A.: The High-risk Mother-Infant Dyad – a Challenge for Nursing." *Nursing Forum,* VI:1:94, 1967.

Slatin, M.: "Extra Protection for High-risk Mothers and Babies." *American Journal of Nursing,* 67:1241, June 1967. (Study of a project in Nebraska; comprehensive preconceptional, prenatal, delivery and postnatal teaching for mothers with the focus on potential or high risk mothers.)

Tiza, V. B., and Gumpertz, E.: "The Parents' Reaction to the Birth and Early Care of Children with Cleft Palate." *Pediatrics,* 30:86, July 1962. (Parents' reactions, anxieties, needs.)

Von Schilling, K. C.: "The Birth of a Defective Child." *Nursing Forum,* VII:4:424, 1968. (Explains what happens to mother of a child who has an abnormality while in the delivery room, post partum unit, and while infant is in nursery.)

Wolff, J. R.: "The Emotional Reaction to a Stillbirth." *American Journal of Obstetrics and Gynecology,* 108:73, September 1, 1970.

OTHER PUBLICATIONS

Abbott Laboratories: *The Human Placenta.* North Chicago, Spring 1956.

Health Services for Mothers and Children – under Title V, Social Security Act. Washington, D.C., U.S. Department of Health, Education and Welfare, 1969.

NOTES

Guide 14

POLLY PAIGE IS ALONE

PART I. POLLY PAIGE'S PRENATAL CARE

Polly Paige, a single 23-year-old fashion editor, has been pregnant for five months. She left her position on a newspaper in her home town two months ago and moved into a furnished two-room apartment in a distant city. The baby's father is presently paying the rent and she receives small weekly financial supplements from her parents which enable her to manage satisfactorily. She had rheumatic fever with an enlarged heart when she was nine years old. She has had no further exacerbations of the rheumatic fever and there have been no restrictions on her activity. Polly says since she became pregnant she has had to give up some of her favorite activities – eating out, going to the movies and dancing. She says she is bored with staying home and watching television all day. The baby's father, Paul, is in the service and she has not seen him since she knew of her pregnancy. She does not know if they will marry.

Polly is being cared for by a private obstetrician to whom she was referred by her family physician.

1. Polly Paige is an unmarried woman expecting a baby. State how your background, attitudes and feelings will influence your relationship with her.

2. There are many stereotyped beliefs about unmarried pregnant women. Identify at least two of these and state how each has influenced health care received by these women.

3. A classmate tells you that almost all unmarried pregnant girls are teenagers.

    a. How frequently do pregnancies occur in unmarried teenagers?

    b. How many babies are born to unmarried mothers in the United States?

    c. How does this compare with 20 years ago? What are some of the factors influencing this trend?

4. Polly's pregnancy is considered high risk.

    a. Why is Polly's pregnancy classified as high risk?

b. What implications does this have for nursing?

5. What community resources might be helpful in assisting Polly to cope with her present situation? What assistance could each of these resources offer?

Polly says she does not wish to talk about "all of the problems" she has been having with her family and her boyfriend since discovering she was pregnant.

6. What are your nursing responsibilities to Polly in terms of helping her cope with her situation?

7. What principles are involved in establishing a trusting relationship with Polly?

8. What is becoming the current philosophy of the medical and nursing professions in relation to the needs and care of the unmarried expectant mother and father?

9. Polly has decided to place her baby for adoption after he is born.

   a. What agencies and resources are available to assist Polly in making arrangements for the adoption?

   b. What are some of the laws regarding rights, custody and responsibilities of the child and the unmarried parents?

   c. Polly has had a difficult time making her decision to place the baby for adoption. What is your nursing role while Polly is making this decision?

10. What are some of the reasons that women, married or unmarried, place their babies for adoption?

11. What are some of the reasons people decide to adopt children?

12. State the difficulties you might anticipate for the:

    a. Woman who decides to place her baby for adoption

    b. Family who decides to adopt and infant

13. State the significance of Polly's history of rheumatic fever in relation to her pregnancy.

14. As the nurse in her community, you will be seeing Polly throughout the remaining four months of her pregnancy.

    a. Identify at least two tentative goals for Polly. These goals should be broad statements based on Polly's nursing needs as you have been able to identify them thus far.
    b. State the rationale for each goal. The rationale should be based on the needs you have identified and the theoretic knowledge you have obtained.
    c. State the nursing activities needed to achieve the goals you have identified.
    d. State the rationale for each of the nursing activities you state.

PART II. POLLY PAIGE'S LABOR AND DELIVERY

Polly is in her forty-third week of pregnancy and has entered the hospital. Her mother is planning to arrive later in the day to be with her daughter.

15. Polly is experiencing primary uterine inertia which will necessitate induction of labor. This is referred to as dystocia.

a. What is dystocia?

b. What are the causes of dystocia?

c. What is uterine inertia?

d. Differentiate between primary and secondary inertia.

16. Polly's labor will be induced

a. What is meant by "induction of labor"?

b. How is labor induced?

c. What are the criteria for inducing labor?

d. When is induction of labor contraindicated?

17. Polly will be receiving oxytocin (Pictocin) by intravenous infusion.

a. What is the action of this medication?

b. State your nursing responsibilites while Polly is receiving this medication.

18. What are the possible effects of Polly's prolonged pregnancy on the fetus?

19. Polly's labor progresses slowly. After several hours you note meconium-stained amniotic fluid and a fetal heart rate of 98 over a 30 minute period.

a. What is the significance of these observations?

b. What is your responsibility at this point?

20. Polly's obstetrician finds it necessary to perform a cesarian section. Polly receives a spinal block anesthesia and a baby boy is delivered.

    a. What are the usual indications for a cesarian section?

    b. What are the nurse's responsibilities in preparing Polly for the operation?

    c. What are the nurses' responsibilities during the operation to:

        1) The obstetrician

        2) Polly

21. Polly has a low cervical section.

    a. What is a low cervical section?

    b. Compare this with the other types of cesarian sections which might be performed.

PART III. POLLY PAIGE'S POSTPARTAL CARE

22. Polly says she does not know if she wants to see the baby. She did not see him after the delivery. What are the pros and cons of Poly's seeing her baby?

23. Will the fact that Polly is not married influence where she will be placed on the postpartum unit? Why?

24. You will be checking Polly's lochia. How will her lochia compare with that of a woman who has had a vaginal delivery?

25. State the nursing care Polly will need because she has had a spinal anesthetic.

26. As you care for Polly, she says, "It was bad enough to have the baby in the first place. Now I have to have an operation. Nothing has gone right for me." She begins to cry.

    a. How do you feel about Polly's statement?

    b. What is your role in working with Polly at this time?

27. Polly asks if she will always need a cesarian section if she has other babies. State the knowledge you need to answer this question.

28. What are your responsibilities in checking the height of Polly's fundus?

29. Polly has a Foley catheter, which you will be responsible for removing.

 a. State your nursing responsibilities:

  1) While the Foley catheter is in place

  2) Following removal of the catheter

REFERENCES

BOOKS

Bergersen, B. S., and Krug, E. E.: *Pharmacology In Nursing.* 11th Ed. St. Louis, The C. V. Mosby Company, 1969.

Bookmiller, M. M., et al.: *Textbook of Obstetrics and Obstetric Nursing.* 5th Ed. Philadelphia, W. B. Saunders Company, 1967.

Bowlby, J.: *Child Care and the Growth of Love,* pp. 119-128. Baltimore, Penguin Books, Inc., 1959. (Adoption; its meaning to the child and the parents.)

Bryant, R. D., and Overland, A. E.: *Obstetric Management and Nursing.* 7th Ed. Philadelphia, F. A. Davis Company, 1964. (Baptism.)

Feldman, F. L., and Scherz, F. H.: *Family Social Welfare,* pp. 63-72. New York, Atherton Press, 1967. (Definitions of family, nuclear and extended families; roles of family members; family tasks; cycle of family life.)

Fitzpatrick, E., et al.: *Maternity Nursing.* 11th Ed. Philadelphia, J. B. Lippincott Company, 1966.

Fuerst, E. V., and Wolff, L.: *Fundamentals of Nursing.* 4th Ed. Philadelphia, J. B. Lippincott Company, 1969.

Kozier, B. B., and DuGas, B. W.: *Fundamentals of Patient Care.* Philadelphia, W. B. Saunders Company, 1967.

Lerch, C.: *Maternity Nursing.* St. Louis, The C. V. Mosby Company, 1970.

Orlando, I. J.: *The Dynamic Nurse-Patient Relationship.* New York, G. P. Putnam's Sons, 1961.

Pohlman, E., and Pohlman, J. M.: *The Psychology of Birth Planning.* Cambridge, Massachusetts, Schenkman Publishing Company, Inc., 1969. (The desire for children; costs of conception; husband-wife relationships; parental roles; unwanted conceptions and parents' feelings; methods of birth planning, psychological aspects of overpopulation.)

Rodman, M. J., and Smith, D. W.: *Pharmacology and Drug Therapy in Nursing.* Philadelphia, J. B. Lippincott Company, 1968.

Shnider, S. M. (Ed.): *Obstetrican Anesthesia – Current Concepts and Practice.* Baltimore, The Williams and Wilkins Company, 1970.

Vincent, C. E.: *Unmarried Mothers.* New York, Free Press of Glencoe, 1964. (Analysis of the socioeconomic, psychological and family backgrounds of unmarried mothers.)

Williams, S. R.: *Nutrition and Diet Therapy.* St. Louis, The C. V. Mosby Company, 1969.

Ziegel, E., and Van Blarcom, C. C.: *Obstetric Nursing.* 5th Ed., pp. 379-412. New York, The Macmillan Company, 1965.

JOURNAL ARTICLES

Apgar, V., and Stickle, G.: "Birth Defects." *Journal of the American Medical Association,* 204:371, April 29, 1968. (Definition and taxonomy; fetal loss; prevalence.)

Auerbach, A. B., and Rabinow, M.: "Parent Education Groups for Unmarried Mothers." *Nursing Outlook,* 14:38, March 1966. (Goals and content for classes for unwed mothers; nurses' feelings about working with unwed women.)

Brandt, M. B.: "Nutrition in Pregnancy." *Clinical Obstetrics and Gynecology,* 6:604, September 1963.

Burgess, L. C.: "The Unmarried Father in Adoption Planning." *Children,* 15:71, March-April 1968.

Carnes, C.: "What's New in Adoption?" *Today's Health,* 45:44, August 1967.

Clark, A. L.: "The Crisis of Adolescent Unwed Motherhood." *American Journal of Nursing,* 67:1465, July 1967.

Daniels, A. M.: "Reaching Unwed Adolescent Mothers." *American Journal of Nursing,* 69:332, February 1969. (Group meetings; includes characteristics of unwed adolescents, their fantasies; birth control; how nurses learned to work with groups.)

Downs, F. S.: "Maternal Stress in Primigravidas as a Factor in the Production of Neonatal Pathology." *Nursing Science,* 2:348, October 1964. (Reviews causes of perinatal morbidity and mortality; report of research to investigate relationship between maternal stress and neonatal pathology.)

Faigel, H. C.: "Unwed Pregnant Adolescents." *Clinical Pediatrics,* 6:281, May 1967. (A synthesis of current viewpoints; excellent bibliography.)

Gold, E. M.: "Identification of the High Risk Fetus." *Clinical Obstetrics and Gynecology,* 11:1069, December 1968. (Assessment of infant mortality and morbidity; criteria for identifying high risk pregnancy and high risk infant; application of criteria.)

Gray, J. W.: "Liaison Nurses Bridge the Care Gap." *Nursing Outlook,* 15:28, May 1967. (Nurses act as liaison for high risk maternity patients between clinics, hospital and community.)

Hallan, M. B.: "Attitudes Toward the Unwed Mother." *Nursing Clinics of North America,* 2:775, December 1967. (Specific attitudes; theories of cause of illegitimacy; criteria for nursing care.)

Herzog, E.: "Unmarried Mothers – the Service Gap Revisited." *Children,* 14:105, May-June 1967. (Service needs and problems.)

Katz, S. N.: "Legal Protections for the Unmarried Mother and Her Child." *Children,* 10:55, March-April 1963.

Knight, E.: "Conferences for Pregnant, Unwed Teen-Agers." *American Journal of Nursing,*65:123, July 1965. (Establishing the conferences; girls' needs, fears, social problems; fathers.)

Lanman, J. T.: "Delays during Reproduction and Their Effects on the Embryo and Fetus." 3. "Delayed Parturition." *New England Journal of Medicine,* 278:1092, May 16, 1968 (p. 1096 – effects of prolonged pregnancy in man).

Larsen, V. L.: "Stresses of the Childbearing Year." *American Journal of Public Health,* 56:32, January 1966. (Stresses during pregnancy, labor and delivery, postpartum and first three months at home.)

McKinley, E.: "Social Implications of Pregnancy." *Clinical Obstetrics and Gynecology,* 6:685, September 1963.

Middleman, R. R.: "A Service Pattern for Helping Unmarried Pregnant Teenagers." *Children,* 17:108, May-June 1970. (Specific tasks used to bridge communication barrier among teenagers and between girls and group leader.)

Nesbitt, R. E. L., and Richard, A. H.: "High-risk Obstetrics." *American Journal of Obstetrics and Gynecology,* 103:972, April 1, 1969.

"Nursing Care by Correspondence." *Nursing Outlook,* 17:50, July 1969. (A nurse's support of an unwed pregnant teenager by letter.)

O'Leary, J. A.: "Cesarean Hysterectomy: A 15 Year Review." *The Journal of Reproductive Medicine,* 4:231, June 1970.

Pannor, R.: "Casework Service for Unmarried Fathers." *Children,* 10:65, March-April 1963. (Working with teenage and older unmarried fathers.)

Platts, H. K.: "Facts Against Impressions: Mothers Seeking to Relinquish Children for Adoption." *Children,* 17:27, January-February 1970. (Characteristics of 1513 mothers.)

"Problems and Management of Postmaturity and Placental Insufficiency." *The Journal of Reproductive Medicine,* 4:77, March 1970. (Symposium related to problems of terminology and management.)

"Reducing Infant Mortality: Suggested Approaches." *Journal of the American Medical Association,* 193:310, July 26, 1965. (Mortality rates; definitions of rates; factors influencing mortality; high risk pregnancies; care needed.)

Rose, P.A.: "The High-risk Mother-Infant Dyad – a Challenge for Nursing." *Nursing Forum,* 6(1):94, 1967.

Slatin, M.: "Extra Protection for High-risk Mothers and Babies." *American Journal of Nursing,* 67:1241, June 1967. (Study of a project in Nebraska; comprehensive preconception, prenatal, delivery and postnatal teaching for mothers with the focus on potential or high risk mothers.)
Sussman, M. B., and Burchinal, L.: "Parental Aid to Married Children: Implications for Family Functioning." *Marriage and Family Living,* 24:320, 1962.
Townsend, J.: "The Unmarried, Pregnant Adolescent's Use of Educational Literature." *Nursing Outlook,* 15:48, August 1967. (Evaluation of materials given to adolescents; bibliography of available references.)
Zimmerman, D. S., and Gohrke, C.: "The Goal-directed Nursing Approach." *American Journal of Nursing,* 70:306, February 1970.

OTHER PUBLICATIONS

Celestine, S. R.: "Nursing Problems in the Care of the Teen-age Unmarried Mother." In *Phases in Human Development: Relevance in Nursing,* pp. 5-12. ANA 1962. Clinical Sessions, 10 Columbus Circle, New York. (Case studies of 17-year-old and 14-year-old; services needed by unwed teenagers.)
Children's Bureau: *Legislation Guides for the Termination of Parental Rights and Responsibilities and the Adoption of Children.* Washington, D.C., U.S. Government Printing Office, U.S. Department of Health, Education and Welfare, 1961.
Children's Bureau: *When You Adopt a Child.* Washington, D.C., U.S. Government Printing Office, U.S. Department of Health, Education and Welfare, 1965.
Choate, R. E., and Gallagher, U. M.: *Unmarried Parents – a Guide for the Development of Services in Public Welfare.* Washington, D.C., U.S. Government Printing Office, U.S. Department of Health, Education and Welfare, 1961.
Health Services for Mothers and Children – under Title V, Social Security Act. Washington, D.C., U.S. Department of Health, Education and Welfare, 1969.
Herzog, E., and Bernstein, R.: *Health Services for Unmarried Mothers.* Children's Bureau Publication 425, Washington, D.C., U.S. Government Printing Office, U.S. Department of Health, Education and Welfare, 1964.
Howard, M.: *Multiservice Programs for Pregnant School Girls.* Children's Bureau, Washington, D.C., U.S. Government Printing Office, U.S. Department of Health, Education and Welfare, 1968.
Irelan, L. M. (Ed.): *Low-Income Life Styles.* Washington, D.C., U.S. Department of Health, Education and Welfare, 1967. (Goals and values; life themes; family patterns; education; health practices.)

NOTES

Guide 15

YVONNE YUNG IS A TEENAGER

PART I. YVONNE YUNG'S PRENATAL CARE

Mrs. Yvonne Yung, a petite 16½-year-old, and her 19-year-old husband, Yale, are expecting their first baby in five and one-half months. Yale is currently working for the city newspaper and earns $65.00 a week. He has graduated from high school and hopes to eventually attend the junior college in his community. The Yungs, who have been married six months, live in one side of a duplex; the other side is occupied by Yvonne's mother and three younger siblings. The Yung's rent is $45.00 a month. They frequently eat with Yvonne's family.

Yvonne is receiving her prenatal care at the neighborhood clinic three blocks from her home.

1. Yvonne's pregnancy is considered high risk.

   a. Why is Yvonne's pregnancy classified as high risk?

   b. What implications does this have for nursing?

2. Yvonne makes several comments during your initial prenatal interview, when she is four and one-half months pregnant. Each of these comments has implications for nursing intervention. For each comment, state:

   a. Whether or not additional information is needed from Yvonne

b. The additional information you wish to have (if appropriate)

c. The nursing intervention which is appropriate

1) "I have never had my insides looked at before. Does it hurt?"

2) "I guess babies just come. I don't know how they get here. Yale might, though."

3) "Will I get big and fat while I'm pregnant?"

The following information is available after Yvonne's examination is completed:

Weight:	Before pregnancy	– 104 pounds
	Present	– 115 pounds
Height:	5 ft. 1 in.	
BP:	116/82	
Hgb:	10 Gm	
Hct:	30%	
RBC:	3.8 mil	
FHT:	LLQ 152	

3. Yvonne has anemia.

   a. What is the significance of this in terms of Yvonne's health?

   b. What is the significance of this in terms of the health of her fetus?

   c. Yvonne is given an iron preparation to take and is to eat a diet high in iron. She has told you she doesn't "know how to cook much, but it doesn't really matter because we don't eat breakfast and Yale and I usually eat supper at my mother's."

      1) What additional information do you need before you can assist Yvonne with her diet?

2) State the facts you want to be certain Yvonne knows about her:

a) Diet

b) Iron preparation

4. Understanding the developmental tasks of adolescence is necessary in planning nursing care for Yvonne.

   a. Identify three developmental tasks of the adolescent which may be affected by Yvonne's pregnancy.

   b. State how each of these tasks may be affected by her pregnancy.

   c. State the implications for nursing intervention in assisting Yvonne to cope with these changes related to her developmental tasks.

5. a. Identify two of Yale's developmental tasks which may be altered by Yvonne's pregnancy.

   b. State how these tasks will be effected.

Between Yvonne's third and fourth visits, she has gained eight pounds. Her blood pressure has risen from 116/82 to 140/92. She now has 2+ edema of her legs and her urine shows a trace of albumin. Yvonne is diagnosed as having mild preeclampsia.

6. What is toxemia of pregnancy?

7. Describe the physiological changes which occur in:

   a. Preeclampsia

   b. Eclampsia

8. How do mild and severe eclampsia differ?

9. Yvonne is to have a low-sodium, high-protein diet in addition to her diet high in iron.

   a. Why is this low-sodium, high-protein diet necessary?

b. What facts about this low-sodium, high-protein diet will you want to be certain Yvonne understands?

10. Yvonne has been told that she must have plenty of rest. She spends weekdays baby-sitting for two younger siblings, aged 2 and 3½ years, and her sister-in-law's one-year-old, while their parents work.

    a. State, specifically, how you will help Yvonne plan for more limited activities at home.

    b. What community resources might be able to assist the Yungs? What assistance could they offer?

11. What nursing intervention, in addition to guidance with diet and rest, is indicated because of Yvonne's preeclampsia? Why?

12. If Yvonne should have to be hospitalized because of eclampsia, state the:

   a. Medical intervention usually indicated
   b. Rationale for the medical intervention
   c. Nurse's responsibility to Yvonne
   d. Rationale for the nursing responsibilities

MEDICAL INTERVENTION	*RATIONALE*	*NURSING RESPONSIBILITIES*	*RATIONALE*

PART II. YVONNE YUNG'S LABOR AND DELIVERY

During her thirty-second week of pregnancy, Yvonne arrives at the hospital in labor. When you first see her, she has an anxious expression on her face and speaks very little. Her husband is in the waiting room with Yvonne's mother.

13. What concerns and fears is Yvonne likely to have because of her premature labor?

14. How can you help Yvonne to cope with this situation?

15. What support can you give Yale and Yvonne's mother while they are waiting? Be specific.

16. State how the nursing management of Yvonne's labor will compare with the nursing management of a labor occurring at term.

PART III. YVONNE YUNG'S POSTPARTAL CARE

While you are caring for Yvonne Yung, she asks what you think she did wrong that caused the baby to come so early. "Yale's mother told me I shouldn't have tried to have a baby at my age . . . . You know, the day before the baby came was my birthday. I was 17. I certainly didn't want this kind of birthday present." She begins to cry and says the premature delivery "was all my fault."

Baby Girl Yung is four days old now. Mrs. Yung has not wanted to see her daughter until today.

17. Compare Yvonne Yung's reactions to the birth of her premature infant with reactions of other mothers facing a similar crisis.

18. You are going with Yvonne to see her daughter today.

a. How will you prepare Yvonne for her first visit to the baby?

b. How will you support her while she is in the nursery with her infant?

c. How will you support Yvonne when she returns to her room?

19. State how the nursing management of Yvonne's postpartal period will compare with the nursing management of a mother following a normal spontaneous delivery at term. The birth of Yvonne's infant was spontaneous. Yvonne received no anesthesia during the delivery. She did not have an episiotomy.

REFERENCES

BOOKS

Bergersen, B. S., and Krug, E. E.: *Pharmacology in Nursing.* 11th Ed. St. Louis, The C. V. Mosby Company, 1969.

Callon, H.: "Consultation – a Tool for Helping Mothers." In Bergersen, B. S., et al.: *Current Concepts in Clinical Nursing.* Vol. 2, Chapter 24, St. Louis, The C. V. Mosby Company, 1969. (Nurse's role; self-understanding; understanding mothers and families; objectives of consultation; methods of meeting objectives.)

Cavanagh, D., and Talisman, M. R.: *Prematurity and the Obstetrician.* New York, Appleton-Century-Crofts, Educational Division, Meredith Corporation, 1969.

Duvall, E. M.: *Family Development.* 3rd Ed.Philadelphia, J. B. Lippincott Company, 1971.

Eastman, N. J., and Hellman, L. M.: *Williams Obstetrics.* 12th Ed., pp. 525-560, 715-775. New York, Appleton-Century-Crofts, Inc., 1961.

Fitzpatrick, E., et al.: *Maternity Nursing.* 11th Ed. Philadelphia, J. B. Lippincott Company, 1966.

Group for the Advancement of Psychiatry: *Normal Adolescence: Its Dynamics and Impact,* pp. 27-49. New York, Charles Scribner's Sons, 1968. (Cultural factors in adolescence, with emphasis on western culture and the American middle class.)

Lerch, C.: *Maternity Nursing.* St. Louis, The C. V. Mosby Company, 1970.

Netter, F. H.: *The Ciba Collection of Medical Illustrations.* Vol. 2. *Reproductive System.* New York, Ciba Corporation, 1965.

Nordmark, M. T., and Rohweder, A. W.: *Scientific Foundations of Nursing.* 2nd Ed. Philadelphia, J. B. Lippincott Company, 1967.

Orlando, I. J.: *The Dynamic Nurse-Patient Relationship.* New York, G. P. Putnam's Sons, 1961.

Osofsky, H. J.: *The Pregnant Teen-ager.* Springfield, Illinois, Charles C Thomas, Publisher, 1968. (A medical, social and educational analysis.)

Rodman, M. J., and Smith, D. W.: *Pharmacology and Drug Therapy in Nursing.* Philadelphia, J. B. Lippincott Company, 1968.

Shnider, S. M. (Ed.): *Obstetrical Anesthesia – Current Concepts and Practice.* Baltimore, The Williams and Wilkins Company, 1970.

Spaulding, M. R.: "Adapting Postpartum Teaching to Mother's Low-income Life-styles." In Bergersen, B. S., et al. (Eds.): *Current Concepts in Clinical Nursing.* Vol. 2, pp. 292-297. St. Louis, The C. V. Mosby Company, 1969. (Lower-class behavioral patterns; child care; role of nurse in health teaching.)

Williams, S. R.: *Nutrition and Diet Therapy.* St. Louis, The C. V. Mosby Company, 1969.

JOURNAL ARTICLES

Barnett, C. R., et al.: "Neonatal Separation: The Maternal Side of Interactional Deprivation." *Pediatrics*, 45:197, February 1970. (Pilot study related to changing care of premature infants; significance of neonatal separation: mothers' interaction with their premature infants.)

Battaglia, F. C., et al.: "Obstetric and Pediatric Complications of Juvenile Pregnancy." *Pediatrics*, 32:902, November 1963. (Report of study of 636 pregnancies in girls aged 14 years and younger.)

Brandt, M. B.: "Nutrition in Pregnancy." *Clinical Obstetrics and Gynecology*, 6:604, September 1963.

Clark, A. L.: "The Crisis of Adolescent Unwed Motherhood." *American Journal of Nursing*, 67:1465, July 1967.

Cochran, M. L., and Yeaworth, R. C.: "Ward Meetings for Teen-Age Mothers." *American Journal of Nursing*, 67:1044, May 1967. (Overview and evaluation of group meetings conducted by nurses with young mothers in a hospital maternity unit.)

Conant, L. H.: "Give-and-Take in Home Visits." *American Journal of Nursing*, 65:117, July 1965. (Communication, verbal and non-verbal; patients' and nurses' reactions to home visits.)

Daniels, A. M.: "Reaching Unwed Adolescent Mothers." *American Journal of Nursing*, 69:332, February 1969. (Group meetings; includes characteristics of unwed adolescents, their fantasies; birth control; how nurses learned to work with groups.)

Downs, F. S.: 'Maternal Stress in Primigravidas as a Factor in the Production of Neonatal Pathology." *Nursing Science*, 2:348, October 1964. (Reviews causes of perinatal morbidity and mortality; report of research to investigate relationship between maternal stress and neonatal pathology.)

Engel, G.: "Grief and Grieving." *American Journal of Nursing*, 64:92, September 1964.

Faigel, H. C.: "Unwed Pregnant Adolescents." *Clinical Pediatrics*, 6:281, May 1967. (A synthesis of current viewpoints; excellent bibliography.)

Gimpel, H. S.: "Group Work with Adolescent Girls." *Nursing Outlook*, 16:46, April 1968. (Characteristics of adolescent girls; knowledge needed regarding health, sex, family life; implications for nursing.)

Gold, E. M.: "Identification of the High Risk Fetus." *Clinical Obstetrics and Gynecology*, 11:1069, December 1968. (Assessment of infant mortality and morbidity; criteria for identifying high risk pregnancy and high risk infant; application of criteria.)

Gold, E. M.: "Interconceptional Nutrition." *Journal of the American Dietetic Association*, 55:27, July 1969. (Emphasizes nutritional status of teen-agers and underweight and overweight patients when not pregnant as necessary for healthier babies.)

Goldfarb, A.: "Puberty." *Clinical Obstetrics and Gynecology*, 11:769, September 1968. (Factors modifying onset of puberty; physiology of puberty; progression of puberty.)

Gordis, L., et al: "Adolescent Pregnancy: A Hospital-based Program for Primary Prevention." *American Journal of Public Health*, 58:849, May 1968. (Adolescent family life service program which provides contraceptive informations and services to a selected group of sexually active, nulliparous adolescent girls; discussion groups.)

Gray, J. W.: "Liaison Nurses Bridge the Care Gap." *Nursing Outlook*, 15:28, May 1967. (Nurses act as liaison for high risk maternity patients between clinics, hospital and community.)

Hammar, S. L., and Holterman, V.: "Interviewing and Counseling Adolescent Patients." *Clinical Pediatrics*, 9:47, January 1970.

"Fourteen Institutions Keep Track of 60,000 Infants: Poorly Nourished Mothers – Major Birth Defect Focus." *JAMA Medical News*, 204:24, May 20, 1968.

Israel, S. L., and Woutersz, T. B.: "Teen-age Obstetrics." *American Journal of Obstetrics and Gynecology*, 85:659, 1963.

Iungerich, Z.: "High School for Unwed Mothers." *American Journal of Nursing*, 67:92, January 1967. (How a school nurse works with unmarried pregnant teenagers in a school curriculum designed to help these students continue their education.)

Kariel, P. E.: "Social Class, Age, and Educational Group Differences in Childbirth Information." *Marriage and Family Living*, 25:353, August 1963. (Comparison of knowledge regarding childbirth of primiparas among wives of university students of higher socioeconomic status and the "medically indigent.")

Klaus, M. H., et al.: "Human Maternal Behavior at the First Contact with Her Young." *Pediatrics*, 46:187, August 1970. (Mothers' initial contact with their normal newborn infants and with premature infants in Isolettes.)

Knight, E.: "Conferences for Pregnant, Unwed Teen-Agers." *American Journal of Nursing*, 65:123, July 1965. (Establishing conferences; girls' needs, fears, social problems; fathers.)

Larsen, V. L.: "Stresses of the Childbearing Year." *American Journal of Public Health*, 56:32, January 1966. (Stresses during pregnancy, labor, delivery, postpartum and first three months at home.)

Litchfield, H. R., and Gillman, J. H.: "Effect of Toxemia of Pregnancy on the Newborn." *Medical Times*, 94:933, August 1966.

McGanity, W. J., et al.: "Pregnancy in the Adolescent, 1. Preliminary Summary of Health Status." *American Journal of Obstetrics and Gynecology*, 103:773, March 15, 1969. (Obstetric, socioeconomic, educational, nutritional and biochemical information regarding 800 adolescents. Implications for educational, social and health – including nutrition – preparation.)

McMurray, G. L.: "Continuing Education for Teenage Parents." *Nursing Outlook*, 17:66, December 1969. (Providing education in the schools to help teenagers become adequate parents and breadwinners.)

Mason, E. A.: "Method of Predicting Crisis Outcome for Mothers of Premature Babies." *Public Health Research,* 78:1031, December 1963. (Study of 86 mothers who delivered prematurely; characteristics of those who had good and poor outcomes to the stress. Implications for guidance.)

Middleman, R. R.: "Service Pattern for Helping Unmarried Pregnant Teenagers." *Children,* 17:108, May-June 1970. (Specific tasks used to bridge communication barrier among teenagers and between girls and group leader.)

Nesbitt, R. E. L.: "Primary Prevention from the Viewpoint of the Obstetrician." In Lytle, N. A.: *Maternal Health Nursing,* pp. 31-49. Dubuque, Iowa, William C. Brown Company, Inc., 1967. (Prenatal care; prematurity; third trimester bleeding; fetal distress; toxemia; labor.)

Nesbitt, R. E. L., and Richard, A. H.: "High Risk Obstetrics." *American Journal of Obstetrics and Gynecology,* 103:972, April 1, 1969.

Osofsky, H. J.: "Somatic, Hormonal Changes during Adolescence." *Hospital Topics,* 46:95, April 1968. (Somatic and hormonal changes, including primary and secondary changes, menarche, pathological causes of menstrual irregularity.)

Owens, C.: "Parents' Response to Premature Birth." *American Journal of Nursing,* 60:1113, August 1960. (Case presentations of two families' very different responses. The premature birth, hospitalization and adjustments at home; reactions of 18-month-old siblings.)

"Reducing Infant Mortality: Suggested Approaches." *Journal of the American Medical Association,* 193:310, July 26, 1965. (Mortality rates; definitions of rates; factors influencing mortality; high risk pregnancies; care needed.)

"Robischon, P.: "The Challenge of Crisis Theory for Nursing." *Nursing Outlook,* 15:28, July 1967. (Types of crises – developmental and situational; includes birth of an atypical child; parenthood; general principles applicable to crisis intervention.)

Rose, P. A.: The High-risk, Mother-Infant Dyad – a Challenge for Nursing." *Nursing Forum,* 6(1):94, 1967.

Semmens, J. P.: "Fourteen Thousand Teen-age Pregnancies." *American Journal of Nursing,* 66:308, February 1966. (Statistical data and information regarding toxemia, weight gain, abortion, prematurity and duration of labor. Implications for specific nursing intervention.)

Shank, R. E.: "A Chink in Our Armour." *Nutrition Today,* 5:2, Summer 1970. (Guidelines for new approach to dietary management of pregnancy, including adolescents, anemia, toxemias.)

Slatin, M.: "Extra Protection for High-risk Mothers and Babies." *American Journal of Nursing,* 67:1241, June 1967. (Study of a project in Nebraska; comprehensive preconception, prenatal, delivery and postnatal teaching for mothers, with the focus on potential or high risk mothers.)

Sussman, M. B., and Burchinal, L.: "Parental Aid to Married Children: Implications for Family Functioning." *Marriage and Family Living,* 24:320, 1962.

Townsend, J.: The Unmarried, Pregnant Adolescent's Use of Educational Literature." *Nursing Outlook,* 15:48, August 1967. (Evaluation of materials given to adolescents; bibliography of available references.)

Watkins, E. L.: "Low-income Negro Mothers – Their Decision to Seek Prenatal Care." *American Journal of Public Health,* 58:655, April 1968. (Emphasizes need for comprehensive maternity programs and concern for the individual.)

OTHER PUBLICATIONS

Cahill, I. D.: "The Mother from the Slum Neighborhood." *Conference on Maternal and Child Nursing: Current Concepts in Nursing Care,* Columbus, Ohio, Ross Laboratories, 1964.

Celestine, Sr.: "Nursing Problems in the Care of the Teen-age Unmarried Mother." In *Phases in Human Development: Relevance in Nursing,* pp. 5-12. ANA 1962. Clinical Sessions, 10 Columbus Circle, New York. (Case studies of 17-year-old and 14-year-old; services needed by unwed teenagers.)

Children's Bureau: *The Adolescent in Your Family.* Washington, D.C., U.S. Department of Health, Education and Welfare, 1967.

Health Services for Mothers and Children – under Title V, Social Security Act. Washington, D.C., U.S. Department of Health, Education and Welfare, 1969.

Ross Laboratories: *The Adolescent Unwed Mother.* Columbus, Ohio, 1965. (Round table discussion: facts and fallacies; emotional impact; services; medical management; nursing needs.)

Runnerstrom, L.: "Food Iron Intake and Hemoglobin Levels in Uncomplicated Pregnancy: Implications for Nursing." *Clinical Sessions,* Number 11, pp. 28-30. American Nurses Association, 1964.

NOTES

Guide 16

THE YUNGS' INFANT IS PREMATURE

Baby Girl Yung, age 1 hour, is a 3-pound, 5-ounce (1500-gram), 16-inch (40-centimeter) premature infant born after 32 weeks gestation. She is the first child of Yvonne and Yale Yung. Mrs. Yung, 17 years old, developed mild preeclampsia during her sixth month of pregnancy. Baby Girl Yung's Apgar score at 1 minute was 1 (heart 1, respiration 0, color 0, reflex irritability 0, muscle tone 0). She was resuscitated, placed in an Isolette with high humidity and oxygen and transferred to the premature intensive care nursery. Mrs. Yung was awake at the time of the baby's spontaneous delivery.

1. Baby Girl Yung is a premature infant.

   a. State the criteria for classifying an infant as premature.

   b. What information from Mrs. Yung's history would have lead one to suspect the possibility of prematurity?

c. Differentiate between the terms premature, immature, low-birth weight, and small-for-date, which are used in the literature.

d. What are the causes of prematurity?

e. What are the causes of death in premature infants?

2. What is the significance of Baby Girl Yung's Apgar score of 1?

3. What immediate nursing care will you be prepared to give Baby Girl Yung when she arrives in the nursery?

4. In order to care for Baby Girl Yung effectively, you need to understand her anatomical, physiological and biochemical characteristics. These characteristics are frequently referred to as handicaps of the premature infant. Using this modified infant assessment form, state the characteristics you would expect to see when assessing Baby Girl Yung.

GENERAL CHARACTERISTICS

Skin

color

desquamation

lanugo

vernix caseosa

rashes

tactile sense

General body proportions

head to body

head circumference to chest circumference

length

weight

Behavior

motor activity when awake

muscle tone

Reflexes

- tonic neck
- Moro
- Step (dance) if held upright
- neck-righting

Head

- caput succedaneum
- ears: position, formation, hearing
- general characteristics

Face

- symmetry
- milia
- eyes (blink; color; reaction to light; subconjunctival hemorrhage; strabismus)
- rooting reflex
- mouth (mouthing; sucking reflex; swallowing reflex; sucking pads)

Cry: character

Chest

- respirations (rate, character)

heart rate and rhythm

breast tissue

breast engorgement

circumference

Extremities

symmetry of size and movement

peripheral circulation

hands and feet

development of finger and toe nails

grasp reflex

Babinski reflex

creases of feet

Abdomen

shape

symmetry

umbilical cord: number of vessels

Genitalia

edema

vaginal discharge

vaginal tag

testes

CHARACTERISTICS OF INFANT WHEN PRONE

Neck: ability to support head

Extremities: swimming reflex

5. Baby Girl Yung is placed in an Isolette with high humidity and oxygen concentrations below 40 per cent.

   a. State her anatomical, physiological and biochemical handicaps which necessitate the use of the Isolette, high humidity and low oxygen concentrations.

   b. State Baby Girl Yung's nursing needs as a result of each of the characteristics you have mentioned.

   c. What are your nursing responsibilities in relation to Baby Girl Yung's Isolette?

6. Baby Girl Yung is to have nothing by mouth. When she is ready to begin taking fluids, she will receive small amounts of fluid by gavage every two or three hours.

   a. State her anatomical and physiological handicaps which necessitate small frequent gavage feedings.

   b. How will you know when Baby Girl Yung no longer needs to be fed by gavage?

   c. State the principles you must consider when feeding her by gavage and the nursing implications of each. Include insertion of tube, the actual feeding and removal of the tube. How would this differ if the tube was not removed after each feeding?

7. It is extremely important to protect Baby Girl Yung against infection.

   a. State her physiological and biochemical handicaps which necessitate this protection.

b. How will you provide this protection?

c. What standards are listed by the Academy of Pediatrics regarding the protection of premature infants?

8. a. State any additional physiological handicaps Baby Girl Yung has as a result of her prematurity.
   b. State the nursing care necessitated by each of these handicaps.

When Baby Girl Yung arrived in the nursery, her respirations were 58, pulse 140 and temperature 95.4°F. Within the next few hours, she developed severe respiratory distress with an expiratory grunt, marked inspiratory sternal retractions, "see-saw" respirations of 88 to 94 per minute, flaring of the alae nasi, and cyanosis when in oxygen concentrations below 80 per cent. Her heart rate increased from 166 to 174 beats per minute. Her skin temperature is now 96.2°F. Her body is limp and she is lying supine in a frog-leg position.

Her chest x-ray revealed changes consistent with hyaline membrane syndrome. On examination, fine rales were heard at the base of both lungs, breath sounds were diminished and a dullness to percussion of the chest was noted. A blood sample revealed pO_2 of 66 mm Hg, pCO_2 of 70 mm Hg, arterial pH of 7.21 and potassium of 5.6 mEq.L.

A diagnosis of respiratory distress syndrome was made and an umbilical catheter was inserted. Baby Girl Yung is now receiving 10 per cent glucose and water with sodium bicarbonate at 5 ml per hour. Assisted ventilation has not been necessary, but a respirator is at her bedside in case it is needed. She is receiving prophylactic antibiotics intramuscularly every 12 hours. She is to have nothing by mouth and is to remain in oxygen concentrations sufficient to keep her pink. She requires frequent oropharyngeal suctioning for moderate amounts of clear mucus.

9. What is respiratory distress syndrome?

10. Use the chart below to state the:
    a. Manifestations of the respiratory distress syndrome
    b. Pathophysiology underlying the respiratory distress syndrome
    c. Medical management of the respiratory distress syndrome

MANIFESTATIONS	*PATHOPHYSIOLOGY*	*MEDICAL MANAGEMENT*

11. Baby Girl Yung is retracting and has an expiratory grunt.

   a. Define retractions.

   b. How will you differentiate between mild, moderate and severe retractions?

   c. Differentiate between substernal, suprasternal and intercostal retractions.

   d. Describe her "see-saw" (paradoxical) respirations.

   e. What is an expiratory grunt?

12. Develop a nursing care plan for Baby Girl Yung for 24 hours while she has respiratory distress syndrome by stating the:

   a. Goals for Baby Girl Yung. These goals should be statements based on her nursing needs.

   b. Rationale for each goal. The rationale should be based on her age, condition and therapeutic plan of care.

   c. Nursing activities needed to meet the goals you have identified. These activities should be specific and should include observations to be made.

   d. Rationale for each nursing activity

GOALS	*RATIONALE*	*NURSING ACTIVITIES*	*RATIONALE*

13. Baby Girl Yung is receiving high concentrations of oxygen.

a. What are the latest theories concerning the use of high concentrations of oxygen for premature infants?

b. What is the relationship between oxygen concentrations and retrolentalfibroplasia?

14. While Baby Girl Yung is acutely ill, her father and grandparents spend many hours standing outside the nursery window or pacing in the corridor. Each time you or other nurses look up or leave the nursery, they inquire about the baby's progress. What is your role in relation to Baby Girl Yung's relatives?

Baby Girl Yung, who has been named Yolanda, gradually improves. Her lungs clear, her respiratory distress diminishes, the umbilical catheter is removed and she begins feedings by gavage.

15. Yolanda remained in the Isolette for nearly five weeks before she was transferred to an Armstrong incubator and later to a crib.

    a. Compare the function of an Air-Shields Isolette with that of an Armstrong incubator.

    b. What criteria will be used to determine when Yolanda can be removed from the Isolette?

    c. What meaning does Yolanda's long period in the Isolette have for Yolanda and her mother?

d. What are the current thoughts concerning stimulation and body contact for premature infants?

Once Yolanda has recovered from her respiratory distress and is progressing satisfactorily (about three weeks of age), you begin helping the Yungs plan for Yolanda's discharge and care at home.

16. As Yolanda improves, the Yungs wonder whether she will be normal. State the knowledge you need about the growth and development of premature infants in order to discuss this with the Yungs.

17. State the information which is needed by the Yungs prior to Yolanda's discharge.

18. What health-related personnel may be helpful to the Yungs while Yolanda is hospitalized and when she returns home? What would be their possible roles in working with this family?

REFERENCES

BOOKS

American Academy of Pediatrics: *Standards and Recommendations for Hospital Care of Newborn Infants.* Evanston, Illinois, 1964.

Babson, S. G., and Benson, R. C.: *Primer on Prematurity and High-risk Pregnancy.* St. Louis, The C. V. Mosby Company, 1966. (Definitions; causes; nursing care; hospital; preparation for discharge; physiological handicaps; sequelae; prevention.)

Bergersen, B. S., and Krug, E. E.: *Pharmacology in Nursing.* 11th Ed. St. Louis, The C. V. Mosby Company, 1969.

Blake, F. C., et al.: *Nursing Care of Children.* 8th Ed. Philadelphia, J. B. Lippincott Company, 1970.

Cavanaugh, D., and Talisman, M. R.: *Prematurity and the Obstetrician.* New York, Appleton-Century-Crofts, Educational Division, Meredith Corporation, 1969.

Crosse, V. M.: *The Premature Baby,* pp. 1-12. Boston, Little, Brown and Company, 1966. (Definitions; characteristics; brief comparison with normal newborn; management and nursing care.)

Drillen, C. M.: *The Growth and Development of the Prematurely Born Infant,* pp. 1-16. Baltimore, The Williams and Wilkins Company, 1964. (Definitions; causes; future of prematures; book report of a study of growth and development of premature infants.)

Duvall, E. M.: *Family Development.* 3rd Ed. Philadelphia, J. B. Lippincott Company, 1971.

Fitzpatrick, E., et al.: *Maternity Nursing.* 11th Ed. Philadelphia, J. B. Lippincott Company, 1966.

Huntingford, P. J., et al. (Eds.): *Perinatal Medicine.* New York, Academic Press, 1969. (Amniotic fluid analysis; prevention, diagnosis and treatment of Rh incapability; electronic fetal heart monitoring; fetal blood sampling; clinical relationships between mother and fetus during labor; resuscitation of newborn; high risk baby; treatment of respiratory disturbances in newborn.)

Leifer, G.: *Principles and Techniques in Pediatric Nursing.* Philadelphia, W. B. Saunders Company, 1965.

Marlow, D. R.: *Textbook of Pediatric Nursing.* 3rd Ed. Philadelphia, W. B. Saunders Company, 1969.

McKilligan, H.: *The First Day of Life: Principles of Neonatal Nursing.* New York, Springer Publishing Company, Inc., 1970.

Rodman, M. J., and Smith, D. W.: *Pharmacology and Drug Therapy in Nursing.* Philadelphia, J. B. Lippincott Company, 1968.

Shepard, K. S.: *Care of the Well Baby.* 2nd Ed. Philadelphia, J. B. Lippincott Company, 1968.

Ziegel, E., and Van Blarcom, C. C.: *Obstetric Nursing.* 5th Ed., pp. 598-636. New York, The Macmillan Company, 1965.

JOURNAL ARTICLES

Avery, M. E., and Hodson, W. A.: "The First Drink Reconsidered." *Journal of Pediatrics,* 68:1008, June 1966. (Factors related to time of first feeding of premature infants.)

Barnett, C. R., et al.: "Neonatal Separation: The Maternal Side of Interactional Deprivation." *Pediatrics,* 45:197, February 1970.

Bascola, E., et al.: "Perinatal and Environmental Factors in Late Neurogenic Sequelae, II. Infants Having Birth Weights from 1500 to 2500 Grams." *American Journal of Diseases of Children,* 112:369, October 1966. (Relationship of perinatal and environmental factors to mental development.)

Battaglia, F. C.: "Recent Advances in Medicine for Newborn Infants." *Journal of Pediatrics,* 71:748, November 1967. (Association of obstetric complications with neonatal problems; treatment of idiopathic respiratory distress syndrome; intrauterine growth retardation; neonatal metabolic complications.)

"Bettering the Odds for Survival." *Medical World News,* 9:42, March 1, 1968.

Callon, H. F.: "The Premature Infant's Nurse." *American Journal of Nursing,* 63:103, February 1963. (Emphasis on working with the premature infant's parents.)

"Categorization by Weight and Gestational Age of the Infant at Birth." *Journal of Pediatrics,* 71:309, August 1967. (Editorial regarding need for new classification.)

Cornblath, M., et al.: "Research and Nursing Care in the Premature Nursery." *American Journal of Nursing,* 62:92, July 1962.

De Hirsch, K., et al.: "Comparisons Between Prematurely and Maturely Born Children at Three Age Levels." *American Journal of Orthopsychiatry,* 36:616, July 1966. (Results of tests administered to premature and mature children of average intelligence at end of kindergarten, first and second grades.)

DeMarco, J. P., and Reed, R.: "Care of the High-risk Infant in the Intensive Care Unit." *Nursing Clinics of North America,* 5:375, September 1970.

Davidson, M., et al.: "Feeding Studies in Low-Birth-Weight Infants." *Journal of Pediatrics,* 70:695, May 1967.

Donnelly, J. F.: "Etiology of Prematurity." *Clinical Obstetrics and Gynecology.* 7:647, September 1964.

Drillien, C. M.: "A Longitudinal Study of the Growth and Development of Prematurely and Maturely Born Children." *Archives of Diseases in Childhood,* 36:1, February 1961. (Physical development age 2-4 years.)

Drillien, C. M.: "A Longitudinal Study of the Growth and Development of Prematurely and Maturely Born Children." *Archives of Diseases in Childhood,* 36:233, June 1961. (Mental development ages two to five years.)

Drillien, C. M.: "The Small-for-Date Infant: Etiology and Prognosis." *Pediatric Clinics of North America,* 17:9, February, 1970. (Etiology; long-term prognosis by intrauterine growth; postnatal malnutrition; associated congenital anomalies; significance of maternal estriol excretion.)

"Drug Hazards to the Premature." *JAMA Medical News,* 203:26, January 29, 1968. (Physiological immaturity; effect of drugs taken by mother during pregnancy and labor.)

Fierer, J., et al.: "Contaminated Resuscitators: Fatal Threat to Newborns." *Hospital Topics,* 44:77, October 1968. (Infection of preemies with *Pseudomonas* – causes and care.)

Gold, E. M.: "Identification of the High Risk Fetus." *Clinical Obstetrics and Gynecology,* 11:1069, December 1968.

Graw, R. W., and De'ak, W. R.: "Respiratory Distress Syndrome." *Clinical Pediatrics,* 7:510, September 1968. (Protocol for management; includes temperature regulation, diagnostic measures, acid-base balance and respirator care.)

James, L. S., et al.: "Respiratory Physiology of the Fetus and Newborn Infant." *New England Journal of Medicine,* 271:1403, December 31, 1964.

"Low Birth Weight – a High Risk Factor?" *JAMA Medical News,* 195:35, January 3, 1966. (Report of follow-up growth and development of 400 premature infants to age 17 years.)

Lubchenco, L. O.: "Assessment of Gestational Age and Development at Birth." *Pediatric Clinics of North America,* 17:125, February 1970. (Obstetric and pediatric clinical estimate; laboratory estimate; morbidity and mortality related to birth weight and gestational age)

McKay, R. J., and Lucey, J. F.: "Neonatology." *The New England Journal of Medicine,* 270:1231, June 4, 1964. (Drugs; immunity; respiratory distress syndrome; infants of diabetic mothers; hypoglycemia.)

McKay, R. J., and Lucey, J. F.: "Neonatology." *The New England Journal of Medicine,* 270:1292, June 11, 1964. (Jaundice; twins; prematurity; aids to diagnosing neonatal diseases.)

Neal, M. V., and Nauen, C. M.: "Ability of Premature Infant to Maintain His Own Body Temperature." *Nursing Research,* 17:396, September-October 1968. (Study of infants weighing between 1450 and 1750 grams; temperature regulation prior to and following removal from incubator.)

"New Parameters in Neonatal Growth – Cell Number and Cell Size." *Journal of Pediatrics,* 71:459, September 1967. (Possibility of cell growth and size in classification of newborns.)

"No More Preemies?" *Clinical Pediatrics,* 7:247, May 1968. (Refers to use of term "premature.")

Pringle, J. A.: "Respiratory Distress Unit." *American Journal of Nursing,* 68:2370, November 1968. (Care of premature infants with respiratory distress; Silverman score for respiratory distress.)

Robinson, N. M., and Robinson, H. B.: "A Follow-up Study of Children of Low Birth Weight and Control Children at School Age." *Pediatrics,* 35:425, March 1965. (Comprehensive follow-up of 227 8 to 10-year-olds; influence of social background significant.)

Rothschild, B. F.: "Incubator Isolation as a Possible Factor to the High Incidence of Emotional Disturbance among Prematurely Born Persons." *Journal of Genetic Psychology,* 110:287, June 1967.

Sinclair, J. C.: "Heat Production and Thermoregulation in the Small-for-Date Infant." *Pediatric Clinics of North America,* 17:147, February 1970. (Heat production and dissipation; physiological responses to heat and cold; clinical consequences of cold stress in small-for-date and full-term infants.)
Sly, R. M.: "Practical Aspects of Infant Feeding." *Clinical Pediatrics,* 2:21, January 1963. (Economy and efficiency techniques of formula preparation; feeding cold formula to premature infants.)
Torrance, J. T.: "Temperature Readings of Premature Infants." *Nursing Research,* 17:312, July-August 1968. (Comparison of axillary and rectal temperatures of premature infants; length of time for temperature to be registered.)
Wessel, M. A.: "Maternal and Child Nursing – as a Pediatrician Sees it." *Nursing Outlook,* 11:207, March 1963.
Wiener, G.: "Correlates of Low Birth Weight: Psychological Status at Six to Seven Years of Age." *Pediatrics,* 35:434, March 1965. (Study of 442 low birth weight children.)
Wortis, H., and Freedman, A. M.: "The Contributions of Social Environment to the Development of Premature Children." *American Journal of Orthopsychiatry,* 35:57, January 1965. (Results of study of preemies of low social class at age 2½ years.)

OTHER PUBLICATIONS

Carnation Company: *Feeding Premature Infants.* Los Angeles, Nutritional Research Department.
Hasselmeyer, E. G.: "The Premature Neonate's Response to Handling." In *Expanding Horizons in Knowledge: Implications for Nursing,* pp. 15-24. ANA 1964 Clinical sessions, 10 Columbus Circle, New York. (Study of 60 premature infants; challenges the practice of minimal handling.)
Health Services for Mothers and Children – under Title V, Social Security Act. Washington, D.C., U.S. Department of Health, Education and Welfare, 1969.
Ross Laboratories, *Currents in Public Health.* Vol. 4, Number 4, Columbus, Ohio, April 1964.

NOTES

Guide 17

NURSING CARE OF NEWBORN INFANTS

The nursery area accommodates 26 infants. The nine infants listed below are in the nursery area with 12 other newborn infants. Refer to this list when answering the questions which follow.

NAME	*AGE*	*BIRTH WEIGHT*	*APGAR SCORE (1 min.)*	*PRESENTATION*	*FEEDING*	*OTHER*	*NURSERY*
1. Dawn, Baby Girl	48 hours	6 lb. 1 oz.	6	Vertex	Bottle	Tremors noted; mother addicted to heroin	
2. Gold, Baby Boy	16 hours	8 lb. 10 oz.	6	Vertex	Breast	Color – jaundiced. Mother Rh negative. Baby Rh positive	
3. Hartman, Baby Girl	48 hours	7 lb.	7	Vertex	Cleft lip feeder (Asepto syringe with rubber tip)	Has cleft lip and cleft palate	
4. Newman, Baby Boy	36 hours	6 lb. 13 oz.	9	Vertex	Bottle	Color – pink	

NAME	*AGE*	*BIRTH WEIGHT*	*APGAR SCORE (1 min.)*	*PRESENTATION*	*FEEDING*	*OTHER*	*NURSERY*
5. Post, Baby Boy	8 days	7 lb. 3 oz.	8	Breech	Bottle	Post mature, Color—jaundiced. Diarrhea	
6. Rubin, Baby Girl	7 days	5 lb. 11 oz.	4	Vertex	Bottle	Has rubella syndrome (congenital heart disease, cataracts). Temperature – 98.8°F.	
7. Sugarman, Baby Girl	3 days	10 lb. 6 oz.	5	Cesarean	Bottle	Color – pale, Mother has diabetes Temperature – 100.2° F.	
8. Twin, Baby Boy	6 days	3 lb. 10 oz.	2	Breech	Dropper	In Isolette. No respiratory distress. Twin sister died of respiratory distress syndrome. Skin temperature – 96.2° F.	
9. Wellman, Baby Boy	3 hours	7 lb. 6 oz.	9	Vertex	Breast	Circumcised in delivery room. Temperature – 95.6° F.	

1. The nursery area has a transition nursery for infants immediately following delivery, an intensive care nursery for premature and ill infants, and a minimal care (regular) nursery.

   a. State the criteria for assigning infants to each of these nurseries.

   b. For each of the nine infants listed above, state the nursery in which the infant would be placed and your rationale for each placement. Put your answer in the righthand column labeled "Nursery."

   c. What other types of newborn nurseries are there? What is the criteria for placing infants in each of these nurseries?

2. Which of these infants would not be considered high risk infants? Why?

3. Is there any need to know the infant's presenting part at birth? Why?

4. State the additional information you need in order to assume the nursing care of these infants. State the rationale for needing this information.

5. State the significance of the following infants' Apgar scores at one minute.

   a. Baby Boy Wellman, Apgar 9

   b. Baby Girl Sugarman, Apgar 5

   c. Baby Boy Twin, Apgar 2

6. It is important for you to be aware of the standards of infant care in the nursery.

   a. Briefly state the standards of infant care which have been set by the Academy of Pediatrics.

   b. Select one standard which is important in terms of nursing care and state how this standard is met.

7. What daily care is needed by normal newborn infants in the nursery? Why?

8. State the nurse's responsibilities when a newborn infant is admitted to the nursery.

9. The following infants are each to be fed by a different method.
   1) Baby Boy Newman – bottle
   2) Baby Boy Twin – dropper (must remain in Isolette for feeding)
   3) Baby Girl Hartman – cleft lip feeder (Asepto syringe with rubber tip)

   Using the chart on page 300, state the principles to be followed and the nursing measures needed to carry out each of these principles when feeding these three infants.

   a. In the left-hand column, list each principle.

   b. In the column under each infant's name, state the nursing measures you will carry out while feeding him or her. Leave a blank space if the principle does not apply to a specific infant.

PRINCIPLES	*BABY BOY NEWMAN (BOTTLE)*	*BABY GIRL HARTMAN (CLEFT LIP FEEDER)*	*BABY BOY TWIN (DROPPER)*

c. State the observations you will make while feeding these infants.

d. Baby Boy Newman regurgitates when you put him into his crib. Differentiate between regurgitation and vomiting.

10. Compare and contrast the nursing care needed by Baby Boy Wellman, Baby Girl Rubin and Baby Boy Twin in relation to maintenance of body temperature.

11. You will be taking Baby Boy Wellman to his mother for his first breast feeding. Briefly state the guidance and information Mrs. Wellman should have concerning:

    a. Position of mother and infant

    b. Beginning the feeding

    c. Ending the feeding

    d. Characteristics of her milk over the next few days

    e. Nursing from one or both breasts at each feeding

    f. Length of nursing time

12. An infant's nutritional requirements are greater than those of an adult.

    a. Why are an infant's requirements higher than those of an adult?

    b. On the chart below, state the average daily requirement of fluids, calories and protein for full-term and premature infants.

	FULL-TERM	*PREMATURE*
Fluid		
Calories		
Protein		

13. The following infants are receiving the feedings listed below:
    Baby Boy Wellman – human milk
    Baby Boy Newman – formula of evaporated milk, water and Karo syrup
    Baby Girl Twin – Similac (Ross Laboratories)
    Baby Boy Post – Nutramigen (Mead Johnson Laboratories)
    Baby Boy Gold – 5 per cent glucose and water

    a. What determines the type of formula an infant receives?

    b. Compare the above feedings in relation to calories, fat, protein and cost. Where applicable, state the indications for use. Use chart on page 303.

	COWS' MILK	HUMAN MILK	SIMILAC	NUTRAMIGEN	5% GLUCOSE AND WATER
Calories per ounce					
Protein					
Fat					
Cost					
Indications for use					

14. The appearance of infants' stools varies.

    a. What influences the appearance of an infant's stools?

    b. Describe the expected appearance of the stools of:

        1) Baby Boy Post

        2) Baby Girl Rubin

3) Baby Girl Sugarman

4) Baby Boy Wellman

c. How will the characteristics of Baby Boy Wellman's stools differ from those of Baby Girl Rubin's stools when he is a week old?

d. What factors influence the number of stools infants usually have per day?

15. Baby Boy Post has diarrhea.

a. Why is diarrhea a serious problem in the newborn infant?

b. What causes diarrhea in a newborn infant?

c. What nursing observations are pertinent for this infant?

d. Briefly identify the nursing measures indicated when a newborn infant has diarrhea.

16. Baby Boy Gold has erythroblastosis fetalis. His Coombs' test was positive and his bilirubin level was 8 mg. per cent at two hours following birth. His mother's antibody titer was markedly elevated one week prior to delivery.

a. Explain the development of erythroblastosis fetalis.

b. State the meaning of the following laboratory tests.

1) Positive Coombs' test

2) Bilirubin of 8 mg per cent at two hours

3) Mother's elevated antibody titer

c. The following methods are currently used to prevent or treat erythroblastosis fetalis. For each of the therapies listed on page 306, state:

1) Its action (how it prevents or interferes with the development of erythroblastosis)

2) To whom it is given (mother or baby)

3) The indications for its use

THERAPY	*ACTION*	*TO WHOM* *MOTHER*	*BABY*	*USE*
Fetal exchange transfusion				
Newborn exchange transfusion				
Phenobarbital administration				
Phototherapy				
RhoGAM administration				

d. State the nursing observations you will make while caring for Baby Boy Gold regardless of the therapy he is receiving.

17. Why might Baby Boy Hope be jaundiced?

18. Baby Girl Sugarman's mother has diabetes.

   a. What is the significance of this in terms of Baby Sugarman?

   b. State the observations of the baby necessitated by her mother's diabetes.

   c. State the nursing care needed by Baby Girl Sugarman because of her mother's diabetes.

19. Baby Girl Sugarman has a temperature of 100.2° F., which may be a transitory fever of the newborn.

   a. What is the cause of transitory fever of the newborn?

   b. When does this fever occur?

   c. What are your nursing responsibilities as a result of her elevated temperature?

20. Baby Boy Twin is scheduled to have blood drawn to test for phenylketonuria (PKU).

    a. Briefly describe phenylketonuria.

    b. How is PKU treated?

    c. Why is it necessary to wait until Baby Boy Twin has been receiving formula before testing for PKU?

21. Baby Girl Dawn's mother is addicted to heroin.

    a. How does Mrs. Dawn's addiction affect her infant daughter?

    b. What changes in Baby Girl Dawn's behavior will indicate withdrawal symptoms?

    c. How will Baby Girl Dawn be treated if she has withdrawal symptoms?

22. Baby Girl Rubin has rubella syndrome

    a. Briefly describe the rubella syndrome.

b. State the nursing care necessitated by Baby Girl Rubin's rubella syndrome.

23. Briefly state the nursing needs of Baby Boy Wellman.

REFERENCES

BOOKS

Bookmiller, M. M., et al.: *Textbook of Obstetrics and Obstetric Nursing.* 5th Ed. Philadelphia, W. B. Saunders Company, 1967.

Fitzpatrick, E., et al.: *Maternity Nursing.* 11th Ed. Philadelphia, J. B. Lippincott Company, 1966.

Ziegel, E., and Van Blarcom, C. C.: *Obstetric Nursing.* 5th Ed., pp. 640-702. New York, The Macmillan Company, 1965.

JOURNAL ARTICLES

Behrman, R. E., and Fisher, D. E.: "Phenobarbital for Neonatal Jaundice." *The Journal of Pediatrics,* 76:945, June 1970. (Treatment before and after birth.)

Behrman, R. E., and Hsia, D. Y. Y.: "Summary of a Symposium on Phototherapy for Hyperbilirubinemia." *The Journal of Pediatrics,* 75:718, October 1969. (Effects of light; untoward effects; use; guidelines for administration.)

Bowes, W. A., et al.: "Amniocentesis and Intrauterine Fetal Transfusion in Erythroblastosis." *American Journal of Obstetrics and Gynecology,* 93:822, November 15, 1965. (Procedure; results.)

Buchanan-Davidson, D. J.: "Erythroblastosis Neonatorum." *American Journal of Nursing,* 64:110, April 1964. (Reviews antigen-antibody reaction; characteristics and treatment.)

DeMarco, J. P., and Reed, R.: "Care of the High-risk Infant in the Intensive Care Unit." *Nursing Clinics of North America,* 5:375, September 1970.

Fleming, J. W.: "Recognizing the Newborn Addict." *American Journal of Nursing,* 65:83, January 1965.

Freda, V. J.: "The Rh Problem in Obstetrics and a New Concept of its Management Using Amniocentesis and Spectrophotometric Scanning of Amniotic Fluid." *American Journal of Obstetrics and Gynecology,* 92:341, June 1, 1965. (Pathogenesis of erythroblastosis; antepartal management; interpretation of findings.)

Garnet, J. D.: "Pregnancy in Women with Diabetes." *American Journal of Nursing,* 69:1900, September 1969. (Overview of management; characteristics of newborn infant.)

Gautefald, B. T.: "Measures for Controlling Cross-Infection in the Nursery." *Hospital Topics,* 44:111, May 1966. (Causes and control of infection.)

Giunta, F., and Rath, J.: "Effect of Environmental Illumination in Prevention of Hyperbilirubinemia of Prematurity." *Pediatrics,* 44:162, August 1965. (Forty-seven babies, unclothed, treated under lights averaging 90 footcandles, and 49 control babies routinely clothed, placed in room with an average of 10 footcandles of light.)

Gotoff, S. P., and Behrman, R. E.: "Neonatal Septicemia." *The Journal of Pediatrics,* 76:142, January 1970. (Incidence; causes; diagnosis and treatment.)

Gregg, G. S., and Hutchinson, D. L.: "Developmental Characteristics of Infants Surviving Fetal Transfusion." *Journal of the American Medical Association,* 209:1059, August 1969. (Children now nine to 38 months of age.)

Hill, R. M., and Desmond, M. M.: "Management of the Narcotic Withdrawal Syndrome in the Neonate." *Pediatric Clinics of North America,* 10:67, 1963.

Kleiger, J. A.: "The Rh Factor: Past, Present and Future." *Medical Clinics of North America,* 53:1063, September 1969. (Blood groups; erythroblastosis fetalis; amniocentesis; intrauterine transfusion, RhoGAM.)

Lester, R., and Troxler, R. F.: "New Light on Neonatal Jaundice." *New England Journal of Medicine,* 280:779, April 3, 1969. (Effect of phototherapy on bilirubin.)

Lin-Fu, J. S.: "New Hope for Babies of Rh Negative Mothers." *Children,* 16:23, January-February 1969. (Explains Rh factor; hemolytic disease and research studies regarding prevention with Rh immunoglobulin.)

Lucey, J. F.: "Says Benefits of Phototherapy Outweigh Theoretical Risks." *Hospital Topics,* 48:69, January 1970. (Use of phototherapy for neonatal jaundice.)

Lucey, J. F., et al.: "Prevention of Hyperbilirubinemia of Prematurity by Phototherapy." *Pediatrics,* 41:1047, June 1968.

MacDonald, M.: "Intensive Care of the Newborn." *Hospital Topics,* 43:97, July 1965. (Nurses' role in newborn intensive care unit – preemies; newborns with disease or abnormalities.)

Murray, B. L.: "Nursery Planning: Contribution of the Nurse to Design." *Hospital Topics,* 43:112, August 1965. (Nurses' role in planning related to new philosophies and goals regarding family-centered care.)

"Neonatal Exchange Transfusion: Present Status." *Clinical Pediatrics,* 7:125, March 1968. (Indications; route; blood; technique.)

Oliver, H. T.: "Construction of Orthodontic Appliances for the Treatment of Newborn Infants with Clefts of the Lip and Palate." *American Journal of Orthodontics,* 56:468, November 1969.

"Phototherapy and Hyperbilirubinemia." *Journal of Pediatrics,* 74:989, June 1969. (Current status of phototherapy.)

Pollack, W., et al.: "Results of Clinical Trials of RhoGAM in Women." *Transfusion,* 8:151, May-June 1968.

Queenan, J. T.: "Intra-uterine Transfusion for Erythroblastosis Fetal." *American Journal of Nursing,* 65:68, August 1965. (Rationale and indications for fetal transfusion; risks; description of procedure.)

Queenan, J. T.: "Intrauterine Transfusion." *American Journal of Obstetrics and Gynecology,* 104:397, June 1, 1969. (Reviews indications, efficacy criteria, time and complications.)

"Screening of Newborn Infants for Metabolic Disease." *Pediatrics,* 35:499, March 1965.

Thompson, L. R.: "Nursery Infections: Apparent and Inapparent." *American Journal of Nursing,* 65:80, November 1965. (Describes the more prevalent and dangerous organisms; recommendations for a safe nursery.)

Yaffe, S. J.: "Reports Results with Phenobarbital in Treating Neonatal Jaundice." *Hospital Topics,* 48:68, January 1970. (Studies regarding use of phenobarbital for neonatal jaundice.)

Wessel, M. A.: "Maternal and Child Nursing – as a Pediatrician Sees it." *Nursing Outlook,* 11:207, March 1963.

OTHER PUBLICATIONS

Children's Bureau: *Neonatal Narcotic Addiction.* Washington, D.C., U.S. Government Printing Office, U.S. Department of Health, Education and Welfare, 1967.

Ross Laboratories: *Problems of Neonatal Intensive Care Units.* Columbus, Ohio, 1969. (Artificial respiration; catheterization of umbilical vessel; pulmonary oxygen toxicity; gastrostomy feeding for premature infants; prolonged nasotracheal intubation; infection.)

"Treating Hyperbilirubinemia with Phototherapy." *Pediatric Currents,* 19:18, March 1970. (Guidelines for use of phototherapy.)

NOTES

Guide 18

THE NEW FAMILY AT HOME

PART I. AMY, HAROLD AND DAVID WONDER

Amy and Harold Wonder are the proud parents of their first child, David, who was born four days ago following an uncomplicated pregnancy, labor and delivery. Amy's mother will be staying with the Wonders for about two weeks.

David, fed just before leaving the hospital, is asleep when they arrive home. Amy is tired and her mother suggests she take a nap. As soon as Amy gets into bed, David begins to cry. Mrs. Able, Amy's mother, changes his diaper and brings him into Amy to breast feed. After he is fed and asleep, Amy again tries to take a nap. This time the doorbell rings and three neighbors come to see the new baby. Amy sleeps for an hour after they leave.

David begins to cry for his feeding just as the family sits down to dinner. He is fussy and does not seem to take very much of his feeding. He does not fall asleep as he had been doing in the hospital and remains fretful for nearly three hours. Amy, Harold and Mrs. Able take turns holding him while the others eat. By 10 o'clock the family is exhausted and ready for bed. Amy decides to stay up until David's next feeding because she is sure he will awaken soon. He wakes up at midnight and startles Amy, who had fallen asleep on the sofa. David falls asleep immediately after this feeding. Harold is up at 7 A.M. to get ready for work and Amy remains in bed until David awakens at 7:30.

The next days are very hectic for Amy. Visitors are in and out throughout the days and evenings. David remains awake and fussy each evening for three or four hours. Mrs. Able, neighbors and relatives offer the Wonders many suggestions for managing this situation. Amy continues to be tired and says that her "stitches" are uncomfortable. She is concerned about her ability to care for the baby, especially since he does not seem to be getting as much sleep each day as the books and friends say he should have.

You visit Amy in her home at the end of this first week and note that Amy is tired, uncomfortable and depressed.

1. Identify the factors in Amy's situation at home contributing to her current feelings of being tired, uncomfortable and depressed.

2. What suggestions can you give the family to help them cope with this situation? State your rationale for these suggestions.

3. What is the nurse's role in helping new families plan for and adjust to their new roles following the birth of a baby?

4. Amy's mother, relatives and friends have been giving the Wonders advice about the baby's care. Some of this advice is contrary to that which Amy has learned or read. What can the nurse do to guide and support Amy in relation to this problem?

5. Amy purchased a layette for David several weeks prior to his birth. State the factors Amy needed to consider in selecting clothing for her infant.

6. Amy had questioned the advisability of using a diaper service.

   a. What are the advantages and disadvantages of such a service?

   b. How much does diaper service cost?

c. What are the advantages and disadvantages of cloth and disposable diapers?

7. What factors need to be considered by Amy in determining how much and what type of equipment to purchase for the baby's:

a. Bath

b. Formula preparation

8. What basic furniture and equipment does Amy need for the baby's daily care?

9. How could Amy improvise some of this needed equipment if she does not wish to purchase it?

10. What is the price range for baby clothing, furniture and equipment?

11. Amy is thinking of buying some prepackaged formula to use for supplementing David's feedings. What are the advantages and disadvantages of these formulas?

12. Amy says she thinks David has colic "because he is so fretful." State the facts you need to answer the following questions:

    a. "What is colic?"

    b. "What can I do for him when he gets colic?"

    c. "How can I prevent it?"

13. Amy wants to know how to cut David's tiny fingernails. What suggestions will you give her?

14. Amy has not washed David's head since he has been home because she is afraid of the "soft spot." "I know you told me it was okay to touch, but I'm afraid I'll hurt him."

    a. Why is it necessary for Amy to wash David's head?

b. If David gets cradle cap, how can Amy remove it?

15. When will Amy be able to give David a tub bath?

16. You note a maculo-papular rash on David's perineum in the diaper area.

a. What might David's diaper rash mean to Amy?

b. State some suggestions which might be useful to Amy in:

1) Clearing up the rash

2) Preventing its recurrence

c. There are many products on sale for the treatment of diaper rash. Select three of these products and state the:

1) Action of each ingredient

2) Value of each product in preventing diaper rash

17. Amy asks a number of questions about David's growth and development. State the facts you must have in order to answer these questions.

a. "How much weight should he gain?"

b. "When will he smile?"

c. "For how long will I have to keep burping him?"

d. "When can I take him out in the sun?"

e. "Is there any danger in taking him to the restaurant with us?"

f. "When do babies usually begin getting solid foods?"

g. "I want to have some foods in the house for him. What shall I get?"

h. "In what position should I put him to sleep?"

18. As nurses, we need to be concerned about the future development of the Wonder family.

    a. During David's first year, he will be developing a sense of trust.

        1) State the behaviors of David and his parents which will contribute to his developing sense of trust.

2) State the behaviors of David and his parents which might hinder his developing sense of trust.

3) State the behaviors of David which would indicate that he is:

a) Developing a sense of trust

b) Not developing a sense of trust

b. Select two developmental tasks of the beginning family and state how the nurse can guide the family in accomplishing these tasks.

19. Some babies fail to thrive during their early months of life.

a. What is meant by failure to thrive?

b. What are the characteristics of infants who fail to thrive?

c. What are the characteristics of mothers whose infants fail to thrive?

d. What is the nurse's role in:

1) Preventing failure to thrive

2) Helping the family whose child fails to thrive

20. Amy and Harold do not have other children at the present time. They hope to have other children in the future and will then be faced with preparing David for the birth of a sibling.

    a. How might they prepare David when he is two and a half years old for the birth of a sibling?

    b. How might they prepare David when he is six years old for the birth of a sibling?

PART II. YVONNE, YALE AND YOLANDA YUNG

The Yungs' premature infant weighed 3 pounds, 5 ounces (1500 grams) at birth and plans are being made for her hospital discharge when she weighs 5 pounds. It is estimated their infant, Yolanda, will be in the hospital approximately six weeks. Seventeen-year-old Yvonne and her 19-year-old husband will be at home for this length of time without their infant.

21. What feelings and concerns may the Yungs have while their infant remains in the hospital?

22. How can the nurse in the community assist the Yungs before they are able to bring their baby home?

23. What are the responsibilities of the nursery nurse to the Yungs and their infant daughter, Yolanda?

24. Compare the needs of Yolanda Yung when she arrives home with the needs of a healthy newborn infant who is able to go home when her mother leaves the hospital.

25. Outline the knowledge needed by the Yungs about their infant's care when she comes home.

26. What assistance can the community health nurse provide the Yungs once the baby comes home?

27. Yvonne Yung says she is afraid to bathe or handle the infant because she is so tiny. How can you help Yvonne develop self-confidence in her mothering abilities?

28. The Yungs are teenagers who have an infant daughter. Look at the developmental tasks for infants, adolescents and beginning families. Select one task from each of these areas and state the effect the task will have on the other two tasks you have identified.

   a. List the three tasks you have selected.

   b. How does the task of the infant influence the tasks of the adolescent and the beginning family you have identified? What implications does this have for nursing?

c. How does the task of the adolescent influence the tasks of the infant and the beginning family? What implications does this have for nursing? Remember, there are two adolescents in this family.

d. How does the task of the beginning family which you have selected influence development of the tasks of the infant and the adolescent? What implications does this have for nursing?

29. The Yungs wonder if the baby will "be sick a lot because she is so small."

    a. What knowledge about premature infants is it important for the Yungs to understand?

    b. What well baby care will Yolanda need over the next several months?

PART III. ALICE AND ALLEN AIKEN ADOPT AN INFANT

Alice and Allen Aiken have been married for eight years. They are both 30 years old and have been unable to have a child. Twelve months ago, the couple applied to a social service agency to adopt a baby. They met the requirements of the agency and have been notified that they would have their baby within about six weeks. With the assistance of the agency social worker, they purchased the items they would need in caring for the infant.

Two days ago they were notified that the baby had been born and was in the county hospital. They could see the baby and could plan on taking him home in three days when he would be six days old. The Aikens were very excited about the baby but also apprehensive about caring for their new family member. The social worker accompanied them to the hospital to see the baby on their initial visit.

30. What are some of the legal requirements for adoption which the Aikens probably had to meet?

31. What information can the social worker give the Aikens about the infant so that they will be informed about his history?

32. What information can the nursery nurse share with the Aikens about the baby since his birth to indicate that he is a normal, healthy baby?

33. What questions can you anticipate the Aikens will have about their new baby and his care?

34. Outline the information about baby care you would want the Aikens to know when they assume the care of their new infant.

35. Although prospective adoptive parents may take a newborn baby home, there is often a waiting period before the adoption can become final.

   a. What is the purpose of this waiting period?

   b. What significance might this waiting period have for the Aikens?

36. Why do the names of the infant's mother and father and prospective adoptive parents remain confidential?

37. How would the Aikens' adjustment period of having a new baby at home compare with the adjustment period of a family such as the Wonders?

38. What are the legal rights of the adopted baby?

39. How would the Aikens' attainment of the new family's developmental tasks compare with the attainment of these same tasks by a family such as the Wonders?

REFERENCES

BOOKS

Anthony, E. J., and Benedek, T. (Eds.): *Parenthood: Its Psychology and Psychopathology,* pp. 353-371. Boston, Little, Brown and Company, 1970. (Adoptive parents.)

Auerbach, A. B.: *Parents Learn Through Discussion: Principles and Practices of Parent Group Education,* pp. 201-205. New York, John Wiley and Sons, Inc., 1968. (Adoptive parents.)

Benson, L.: *Fatherhood: A Sociological Perspective.* New York, Random House, 1968.

Bowlby, J.: *Child Care and the Growth of Love,* pp. 119-128. Baltimore, Penguin Books, Inc., 1959. (Adoption – meaning to child and parents.)

Brazelton, T. B.: *Infants and Mothers Differences in Development.* New York, Delacorte Press, 1969.

Clark, A. L.: *Leadership Technique in Expectant Parent Education.* New York, Springer Publishing Company, Inc., 1962.

Duvall, E. M.: *Family Development.* 3rd Ed. Philadelphia, J. B. Lippincott Company, 1971.

Eastman, N. J., and Russell, K. P.: *Expectant Motherhood.* 5th Ed., revised. Boston, Little, Brown and Company, 1970. (Pregnancy; labor and delivery; postpartum; fetal development; newborn.)

Hurlock, E. B.: *Developmental Psychology.* 3rd Ed. New York, McGraw-Hill Book Company, 1968.

La Leche League International: *The Womanly Art of Breastfeeding.* Franklin Park, Illinois, La Leche League International, 1963.

Lidz, T.: *The Person – His Development Throughout the Life Cycle,* pp. 93-116. New York, Basic Books, Inc., 1968.

Mead, M., and Newton, N.: "Cultural Patterning of Perinatal Behavior." In Richardson, S. A., and Guttmacher, A. F. (Eds.): *Childbearing – its Social and Psychological Aspects,* pp. 142-244. Baltimore, The Williams and Wilkins Company, 1967.

Nordmark, M. T., and Rohweder, A. W.: *Scientific Foundations of Nursing.* 2nd Ed. Philadelphia, J. B. Lippincott Company, 1967.

Spock, B.: *Baby and Child Care.* New York, Meredith, 1968.

Stone, L. J., and Church, J.: *Childhood and Adolescence.* 2nd Ed. New York, Random House, 1968.

Vincent, C. E.: *Unmarried Mothers,* pp. 31-51, 181-201, 233-240. New York, The Free Press, 1961. (Attitudes; feelings; rights of participants in adoption.)

JOURNAL ARTICLES

Auerbach, A. B.: "Meeting the Needs of New Mothers." *Children,* 11:223, November-December 1964. (Psychological and social needs of new and expectant parents; implications for care.)

Barbero, G. T., and Shaheen, E.: "Environmental Failure to Thrive: A Clinical Review." *Journal of Pediatrics,* 71:639, November 1967.

Bellam, G.: "The First Year of Life." *American Journal of Nursing,* 69:1244, June 1969. (Reviews fetal development; characteristics of newborn; some development through 12 months.)

Burgess, L. C.: "The Unmarried Father in Adoption Planning." *Children,* 15:71, March-April 1968.

Carner, C.: "What's New in Adoption?" *Today's Health,* 45:44, August 1967.

Chappelear, E. M., and Fried, J. E.: "Helping Adopting Couples Come to Grips with Their New Parental Roles." *Children,* 14:223, November-December 1967. (Discussion groups for adoptive parents.)

Clark, A. L.: "The Adaptation Problems and Patterns of an Expanding Family: The Neonatal Period." *Nursing Forum,* 5(1):92, 1966. (Adaptation to first child and to subsequent children; problems identified; needs of families that are not met.)

Clark, A. L.: "The Beginning Family." *American Journal of Nursing,* 66:802, April 1966. (The phases of establishment, childbearing and childrearing; postpartal needs. Teaching.)

Conant, L. H.: "Give-and-Take in Home Visits." *American Journal of Nursing,* 65:117, July 1965.

Conant, L. H.: "What Helps Mothers to Speak Out." *American Journal of Nursing,* 69:2650, December 1969. (Study of factors influencing interaction patterns in child health conferences.)

Dyer, E. D.: "Parenthood as Crisis: A Re-study." *Marriage and Family Living,* 25:196, May 1963. (Impact of first child on the family; reactions of new mothers and fathers.)

"Economy in Nutrition and Feeding of Infants." *American Journal of Public Health,* 56:1756, October 1966.

Guillot, E. E.: "Patterns of Help for Post-partum Mothers." *Children,* 11:147, July-August 1964. (Summary of assistance for first month postpartum; mothers' comments regarding what they would do next time.)

Hill, L. F.: "Infant Feeding: Historic and Current." *Pediatric Clinics of North America,* 14:255, February 1967.

Hogan, A. I.: "The Role of the Nurse in Meeting the Needs of the New Mother." *Nursing Clinics of North America,* 3:337, June 1968. (Emphasis on mother's need for rest for three to six weeks after baby's birth and need to feel adequate in caring for baby; includes father's needs.)

Katz, S. N.: "Legal Protections for the Unmarried Mother and Her Child." *Children,* 10:55, March-April 1963.

Kay, R. E.: "Toward a Philosophy of Child Rearing." *Clinical Pediatrics,* 7:281, May 1968. (Helping parents develop healthy attitudes.)

Keitel, H. G.: "Preventing Neonatal Diaper Rash." *American Journal of Nursing,* 65:124, May 1965. (Studies of effectiveness of preventing diaper rash with various preparations; hypotheses regarding etiology of rash.)

Larsen, V. L.: "Stresses of the Childbearing Year." *American Journal of Public Health,* 56:32, January 1966.

Newton, N., and Newton, M.: "Mothers' Reactions to Their Newborn Babies." *Journal of the American Medical Association,* 181:206, July 21, 1962. (Factors which may influence reactions; behavior of rejecting and accepting mothers; implications.)

Parmalee, A. H., Jr., et al.: "Infant Sleep Patterns from Birth to 16 Weeks of Age." *Journal of Pediatrics,* 65:576, October 1964. (Records kept by parents of 46 infants.)

"The Prenatal Visit." *Clinical Pediatrics,* 9:309, May 1970. (A letter from a pediatrician to prospective parents recommending a prenatal visit to pediatrician. Comments pro and con these visits.)

Rhymes, J. P.: "Working with Mothers and Babies who Fail to Thrive." *American Journal of Nursing,* 66:1972, September 1966. (Characteristics of mothers; suggestions for nursing intervention.)

Roberts, J. A.: "Immunization: Newborn to School Age." *Applied Therapeutics,* 11:278, May 1969.

Robischon, P., and Scott, D.: "Role Theory and its Application in Family Nursing." *Nursing Outlook,* 17:52, July 1969.

Rubin, R.: "Basic Maternal Behavior." *Nursing Outlook,* 9:683, November 1961. (Mother's behavior toward newborn; identification process.)

Rubin, R.: "Maternity Care in Our Society." *Nursing Outlook,* 11:519, July 1963. (Emphasizes nursing implications regarding what happens to family when mother goes home with new infant.)

Rubin, R.: "The Family-Child Relationship and Nursing Care." *Nursing Outlook,* 12:36, September 1964. (Changing roles and relationships when a new baby is added to the family.)

Rubin, R.: "Food and Feeding." *Nursing Forum,* 6:195, Spring 1967. (Interpersonal relationships.)

Tisza, V. B., and Gumpertz, E.: "The Parents' Reaction to the Birth and Early Care of Children with Cleft Palate." *Pediatrics,* 30:86, July 1962. (Parents' reactions; anxieties; needs.)

Vaughan, V. C.: "A Study of Techniques of Preparation of Formulas for Infant Feeding." *Journal of Pediatrics,* 61:547, October 1962. (Prevalent practices in formula preparation; implications.)

Wessel, M. A.: "Maternal and Child Nursing – as a Pediatrician Sees it." *Nursing Outlook,* 11:207, March 1963.

Weston, J. L.: "Initiating Referrals: A Health Department Approach." *American Journal of Nursing,* 67:332, February 1967. (Informal sessions on maternity ward as initial public health center to provide continuity of care for families.)

Williams, B.: "Sleep Needs during the Maternity Cycle." *Nursing Outlook,* 15:53, February 1967.

OTHER PUBLICATIONS

Branin, V. A.: "A Study of Problems Encountered by Twenty-six Nursing Mothers following Hospital Discharge." *Evaluation of Nursing Intervention,* pp. 13-18. ANA 1964 Clinical Sessions, 10 Columbus Circle, New York. (Seminar for nursing mothers; their experiences and problems; implications for nursing assistance.)

"Children and the Law." *Currents in Public Health.* Columbus, Ohio, Ross Laboratories, March 1962.

Children's Bureau: *Infant Care.* Washington, D.C., U.S. Government Printing Office, U.S. Department of Health, Education and Welfare, 1963.

Children's Bureau: *When You Adopt a Child.* Washington, D.C., U.S. Government Printing Office, U.S. Department of Health, Education and Welfare, 1965.

Children's Bureau: *Your Baby's First Year.* Washington, D.C., U.S. Government Printing Office, U.S. Department of Health, Education and Welfare, 1962.

Ross Laboratories: "Anticipatory Guidance." *Currents in Public Health,* Columbus, Ohio, Vol. 3, Number 4, April 1963.

Ross Laboratories: "The Conflicts of New Mothers." *Currents in Public Health,* Columbus, Ohio, September 1962.

Ross Laboratories: *Discovering Parenthood.* Columbus, Ohio, 1969.

Ross Laboratories: "Problems of Adopted Children." *Feelings,* Columbus, Ohio, October 1962.

NOTES

NOTES

NOTES

NOTES